PITUITARY-OVARIAN ENDOCRINOLOGY

Edited by *Ralph I. Dorfman, Ph.D.,*
Director of Laboratories, Worcester Foundation for Experimental Biology,
Research Professor of Biochemistry, Boston University,
and Professor of Chemistry (Affiliate), Clark University

and *Manuel Neves e Castro, M.D.,*
Attending Endocrinologist and Gynecologist,
Department of Endocrinology, Portuguese Cancer Institute, Lisbon

HOLDEN-DAY, INC., SAN FRANCISCO: 1963

FOREWORD

    This volume is the record of a Symposium on Endocrine Gynecology sponsored by the Portuguese Cancer Institutue in Lisbon in the summer of 1962. It was my pleasure to participate in these discussions and to help in the editing of this volume. The meeting was a huge success and an excellent meeting ground for the discussions of the newer developments in the field of pituitary-ovarian endocrinology, pure and applied.

    This volume outlines most of the important recent advances in endocrine gynecology from aspects of the biochemistry of steroid biosynthesis through new analytical methods which permit a reasonable evaluation of the "androgen burden," some important new reflections on the Stein-Leventhal Syndrome, newer physiological aspects of the gonadotropins, clinical diagnosis and the important advances in sterility and fertility.

    I know that I speak for the visiting American and English contributors when I thank our Portuguese Cancer Institute colleagues, one and all, for their many kindnesses. All of us would hope to have the opportunity in the near future to repay their thoughtfulness and fine hospitality.

Shrewsbury, Massachusetts   *Ralph I. Dorfman*
August, 1963

PREFACE

For anyone devoted to the practice of Gynecology, one of the more fascinating subjects undoubtedly is the study of the hormonal background of gynecological disease. As a matter of fact, gynecologists must be aware of the possible interrelations between diseases of the endocrine glands and the symptoms and signs related to the genital tract. On the other hand, if a clinical endocrinologist wants to have a full picture of a woman under his care, it is not difficult for him to do a vaginal examination or consider for example, an endometrial biopsy.

It is quite understandable that as medical science and technics develop, it becomes increasingly difficult for any one individual to be up to date with the changes that occur almost daily in both specialties. This explains why endocrine gynecology is becoming, in many outstanding medical centers, the field for a new specialty and subject for so many post-graduate courses.

Both from the clinical and the experimental point of view there are obvious interrelationships between endocrinology and gynecology which support the need for specific training in endocrine gynecology and diseases of reproduction. Unfortunately there is not, as yet, a scientific journal concerned with these specific problems.

The present volume has resulted from the kind cooperation of such distinguished authorities as Drs. R. I. Dorfman, R. B. Greenblatt, and J. A. Loraine, who took part in the first Symposium on Endocrine Gynecology which was sponsored in 1962 in Lisbon, by the Portuguese Cancer Institute.

This valuable contribution to medical literature will attract the attention of both endocrinologists and gynecologists to this challenging field.

Lisbon, Portugal   *Manuel Neves e Castro*

CONTRIBUTORS

Bell, E. T.
Clinical Endocrinology Research Unit
Department of Biochemistry
University of Edinburgh
Edinburgh, Scotland

Castro, Manuel Neves e
Department of Endocrinology
Portuguese Cancer Institute
Lisbon, Portugal

Dorfman, Ralph I.
Worcester Foundation for Experimental Biology
Shrewsbury, Massachusetts

Greenblatt, Robert B.
Department of Endocrinology
Medical College of Georgia
Augusta, Georgia

Loraine, John A.
Clinical Endocrinology Research Unit
Department of Biochemistry
University of Edinburgh
Edinburgh, Scotland

Mahesh, Virendra B.
Department of Endocrinology
Medical College of Georgia
Augusta, Georgia

Schmidt-Elmendorff, H.
    Clinical Endocrinology Research Unit
    Department of Biochemistry
    University of Edinburgh
    Edinburgh, Scotland

Neves Da Silva, J.
    Department of Pathology
    Portuguese Cancer Institute
    Lisbon, Portugal

Valle, A. Reis
    Department of Clinical Medicine
    University of Lisbon Medical School
    Hospital St. Maria
    Lisbon, Portugal

TABLE OF CONTENTS

I

Ralph I. Dorfman, Ph.D.
BIOSYNTHESIS AND DETECTION OF ESTROGENS

Considerable new information is now available on the biosynthesis and estimation of estrogens. This chapter will be devoted to a discussion of these areas.

BIOSYNTHESIS OF ESTROGENS

The biological conversion of androgens to estrogens and thus the route of estrogen biosynthesis had been suggested for some years [3, 13, 16, 20], but it remained for radioisotopic technics to establish this interrelationship beyond a reasonable doubt [1, 2, 5, 19]. Specifically, the substrate was testosterone and the products were estrone and estradiol-17β.

Acetate-1-C^{14} could also serve as a precursor for estrone in the pregnant mare [6] but in one study cholesterol did not seem to be a proper intermediate [7]. Contrary to this report, Werbin, et al. [18] demonstrated that cholesterol-4-C^{14} could be converted to labeled estrone by an *in vivo* experiment in a human. The pathway of cholesterol to androgens is well documented and the mechanisms involved in the aromatization of ring A have been elucidated.

Meyer [10] discovered that bovine adrenal glands may hydroxylate androst-4-ene-3, 17-dione at carbon 19, and he suggested that the removal of the C-10 angular methyl group was facilitated by this preliminary oxidation. These reactions had been accomplished by chemical means. The conversion of 19-hydroxy-androst-4-ene-3, 17-dione to estrone by human placental tissue has been demonstrated by Meyer [11], Ryan [15] and Longchampt, et al. [9].

Since the first experiments by Meyer [10], [11] efforts of a number of workers in various laboratories including the Worcester Foundation group have been extended towards the elucidation of the individual steps of estrogen biosynthesis in the human. In *in vitro* work, the term

1

"placenta preparation" was used throughout as the enzyme source
since this tissue is easily available and a good reproducible incubation
system had been established in the pioneer studies of Ryan [15]. It is
expected that all findings with this tissue can be extrapolated to ovarian systems. Innumerable steroid structures were examined with two
aims in mind: (1) to find what compounds could contribute estrogenic
material, even if a very small percentage, to body pools, and (2) to
elucidate the steps in the major pathway of estrogen biosynthesis.

In Table 1-1 are some of the structures which have been tested for
aromatization in ring A by the placental enzyme system. Most of the
compounds were not converted. There were, however, a few which
led to the natural estrogens, estrone and estradiol-17β. 19-Norandrost-
4-ene-3,17-dione was converted in low yield. This substance, which
has been shown to be present in large amounts in mare follicular fluid,
may be a significant source of body estrogens. Androst-4-ene-3, 17-
dione, 19-hydroxyandrost-4-ene-3, 17-dione and 19-oxo-androst-4-
ene-3, 17-dione, as well as testosterone, were excellent substrates.
These are components of the major pathway of biological estrogen
formation. 10β-Carboxy-estr-4-ene-3, 17-dione yielded only a trace
of estrogen and this by virtue of its very rapid decarboxylation to 19-
norandrost-4-ene-3, 17-dione in the presence of placental tissue. Dehydroepiandrosterone yielded estrone in good yield due to its fast oxidation to androst-4-ene-3, 17-dione. Androst-1,4-diene-3, 17-dione
is another source of estrogens; the question of its natural occurrence
in the body is, however, equivocal. Rigorous examination of the uti-
lization of 5α-androst-1-ene-3, 17-dione has been carried out using
C^{14}-labeled substrate. The results show that this compound does not
give rise to phenolic structures.

Secondly, the picture of the major biosynthetic pathway of estrogen
formation from the androgens, androst-4-ene-3, 17-dione and testosterone, is now essentially complete. It has been known for many years
that both the above C_{19}-steroids are transformed to estrogens; many
tracer studies with C^{14}-labeled precursors have been documented. The
next step was the definite establishment of the 19-hydroxylated derivative as an intermediate in the biosynthesis, following up initial experiments where 19-hydroxyandrost-4-ene-3, 17-dione was observed to be
converted to estrone at a faster rate than androst-4-ene-3, 17-dione.
Confirmation of its formation by placental tissue and its transformation, in turn, to estrone was obtained through the isolation of this
oxygenated derivative in incubations with C^{14}-labeled androst-4-ene-
3, 17-dione. The next series of experiments were conducted when
19-oxo-androst-4-ene-3, 17-dione and 10β-carobxy-estr-4-ene-3, 17-
dione became available. The 19-oxo compound was found to be converted even more rapidly than the 19-hydroxy derivative. The carbox-
ylic acid, however, yielded only a trace of estrone, which subsequent
examination revealed arose from its decarboxylated product,

Table 1-1. Conversion of Various Steroids to Estrogens[*]

	Per cent conversion
C_{18}	
19-Norandrost-4-ene-3,17-dione	10
17β-Hydroxy-5α,10β-estran-3-one	0
5α,10α-Estrane-3,17-dione	0
17α-Ethynyl-10β,17β-dihydroxyandrost-4-ene-3,17-dione	0
17α-Ethynyl-17β-hydroxy-19-nor(10β)-androst-5(10)-en-3-one	0
C_{19}	
Androst-4-ene-3,17-dione	40
19-Hydroxyandrost-4-ene-3,17-dione	60
19-Oxo-androst-4-ene-3,17-dione	80
10β-Carboxy-estr-4-ene-3,17-dione	1
17β-Hydroxyandrost-4-en-3-one (testosterone)	40
3β-Hydroxyandrost-5-en-3-one (dehydroepiandro-sterone)	30
Androsta-1,4-diene-3,17-dione	25
5α-Androst-1-ene-3,17-dione	0
1α-Hydroxyandrost-4-ene-3,17-dione	0
1α,3β-Dihydroxyandrost-5-en-17-one	0
1α-Methyl-17β-hydroxyandrost-4-en-3-one	0
2β-Hydroxyandrost-4-ene-3,17-dione	10
2-Hydroxymethylene-17α-methyl-17β-hydroxyandrost-4-en-3-one	0
2βMethyl-17β-hydroxyandrost-4-en-3-one	0
2-Formyl-17α-methyl-17β-hydroxyandrosta-1,4-dien-3-one	0
Androsta-4,6-diene-3,17-dione	0
Androsta-1,4,6-triene-3,17-dione	0
Androst-4-ene-3,11,17-trione	0
11β-Hydroxyandrost-4-ene-3,17-dione	0
11α-Hydroxyandrost-4-ene-3,17-dione	40
6α-Fluoro-17β-hydroxyandrost-4-en-3-one	0
6β-Fluoro-17β-hydroxyandrost-4-en-3-one	0
5α-Androstane-3,17-dione (androsterone)	0
9α-Fluoroandrosta-1,4-diene-3,17-dione	35
17β-Acetoxyandrosta-4,7-dien-3-one	15
C_{21}	
Pregn-4-ene-3,20-dione (progesterone)	0
17α,19,21-Trihydroxypregn-3-ene-3,20-dione	0
6β-Fluoro-16α-methyl-21-acetoxy-11β,17α-dihydroxypregnane-1,4-diene-3,20-dione	0

[*]Gual, et al. [4]

19-norandrost-4-ene-3, 17-dione. Examination of the co-factor requirements for the aromatization of each of the two 19-oxygenated structures above showed that both TPNH and oxygen were essential (Table 1-2).

Table 1-2. Cofactor and Oxygen Requirement for Aromatization[*]

	Gaseous phase	Cofactor	Per cent conversion to estrogen
10β-Carboxy-estr-4-ene-3,17-dione	N_2	DPN	0
"	N_2	TPN	0
"	N_2	–	0
"	Air	TPNH	5
19-Norandrost-4-ene-3,17-dione	Air	TPNH	5
19-Oxo-androst-4-ene-3,17-dione	N_2	DPN	0
"	N_2	TPN	0
"	N_2	–	0
"	Air	TPNH	100
"	"	DPNH	0
"	"	TPN	0
"	N_2	TPNH	5
19-Hydroxyandrost-4-ene-3,17-dione	Air	TPNH	50-60
"	"	TPN	0
"	"	DPNH	0
"	N_2	TPNH	0
Androst-4-ene-3,17-dione	Air	TPNH	30-40
"	N_2	TPNH	0

DPN, DPNH, or TPN (Sigma) 2.5 μMoles; TPNH regenerating system: TPN 2.5 μMoles, gluc-6-P (Sigma) 4.3 μMoles, gluc-6-P dehydrogenase (Sigma) 0.5 K.U.

[*] Morato, et al. [12]

It thus appeared that the sequence of steps from the C_{19}-compounds to the C_{18}-phenols was: androst-4-ene-3, 17-dione →19-hydroxyandrost-4-ene-3, 17-dione →19-oxo-androst-4-ene-3, 17-dione → estrone. Examination of the nature of the 1-carbon moiety, the 19-carbon atom, eliminated in the course of the reaction was next undertaken. Theoretically, via a mechanism of the reverse aldol condensation type, the direct aromatization of the 19-hydroxy structure would yield formaldehyde, and the 19-oxo compound, formic acid. Experimental results obtained can be briefly summarized: when androst-4-ene-3, 17-dione was the substrate, only formaldehyde appeared in measurable quantities;

when 19-hydroxyandrost-4-ene-3, 17-dione was the substrate, both formaldehyde and formic acid appeared; and when 19-oxo-androst-4-ene-3, 17-dione was the substrate, only formic acid appeared. All possible controls of the incubation system and analysis procedures have been run. All blanks were negative. No inter-conversion of formaldehyde and formic acid occurred in the placental system. In no instance was formaldehyde or formic acid formed other than as a product of placental incubations with the steroids above. Steroid fractions were analyzed by paper chromatography. Both estrone and estradiol-17β were always found as products.

It would appear from these results that in the intact animal the following situation may obtain: estrogen can arise from both the 19-hydroxy and 19-oxo structures directly, and it is highly probable that the same enzyme catalyzes the aromatization of both substrates. A provision for the oxidation of the 19-hydroxy function to the 19-oxo grouping is present in the placenta and has been noted. This transformation probably requires TPN, which is always present in this system. It is esthetically pleasing to visualize a situation where TPNH can be internally generated at the site of estrogen formation at the moment when it is needed to catalyze the final step in the biosynthetic sequence. In this respect another source of the reduced or oxidized pyridine nucleotide is in the 17-dehydrogenase reaction which is TPN linked. The biosynthetic steps are summarized in Fig. 1-1. The elucidation of these mechanisms sets the proper stage for studies of control of estrogen biosynthesis under normal and pathological conditions.

DETERMINATION OF PLASMA ESTROGENS

Elegant methods for the determination of estrogens in human urine have been developed and have recently been reviewed [14]. This review also deals with plasma estrogen levels. Of the various plasma methods, however, only two appear to approach the required sensitivity needed to analyze plasma from non-pregnant human subjects. One of these, developed by Svendsen [17], had a sensitivity of about 0.002 μg for estrone and estradiol-17β in plasma. The method is based on the double isotopic derivative principle using S^{35} and I^{131}. Plasma, derived from heparinized blood, is extracted with chloroform and the estrone and estradiol-17β purified, esterified by means of p-iodo-benzenesulphonyl chloride, purification of the esters by paper chromatography and determining radioactivities. Using this method, preliminary plasma values are given for normal women, patients with primary and secondary amenorrhea, and pregnant women.

The second method has been developed in the Worcester Foundation laboratory [8] and is briefly described. Plasma, after adding an

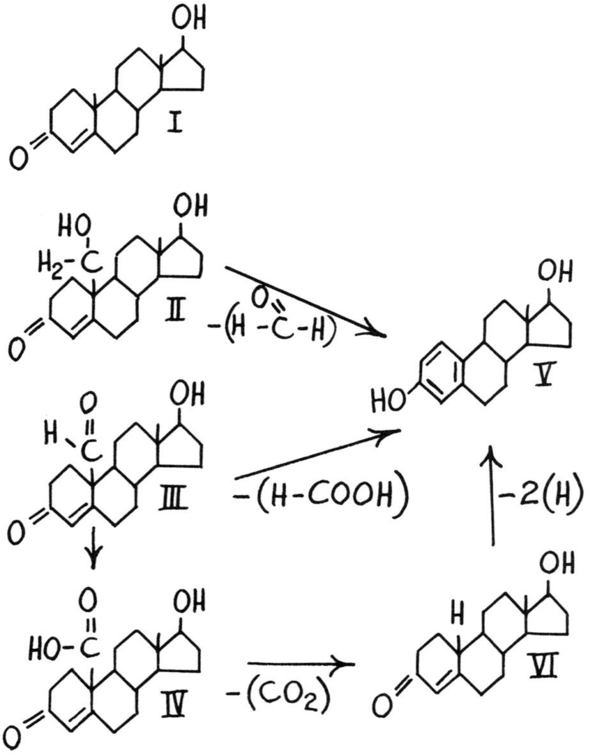

Fig. 1-1. Biosynthesis of Estrogens

I. Testosterone
II. 19-Hydroxytestosterone
III. 19-Oxotestosterone
IV. 10-Carboxy-19-nortestosterone
V. Estradiol-17β
VI. 19-Nortestosterone

insignificant weight but significant number of counts of estrone-6,7-H^3 and estradiol-17β,6,7-H^3, was extracted with a mixture of chloroform: ether (3:1). The residue, after solvent distillation, was dissolved in 70 per cent methanol, placed in a deep freeze overnight, centrifuged, and the supernatant partitioned against petroleum ether. The phenolic material of the 70 per cent methanol fraction was subjected to paper chromatography in the Bush B3 system. The zones containing estrone and estradiol-17β were rechromatographed in the Bush BA and B1 systems, respectively. The quantity of estrogens was determined by a fluorescence method, and the radioactivity (for recovery correction) in a scintillation counter.

The recovery of estradiol-17β and estrone was 62 per cent on a weight basis and 66 per cent on the basis of H^3. The sensitivity of the method using 50 ml of plasma was of the order of 0.002 μg of each of the estrogens.

In a woman studied just at the end of the menstrual flow and at the mid-cycle, about three times as much estrogen was found at the later time (Table 1-3). The mean estrone values for men and women were of the same order in our small number of subjects, but the mean value of 0.031 μg for estradiol-17β for women was considerably higher than the mean value of 0.003 μg for the men. Svendsen [17] reported on

Table 1-3. The Concentration of Estrone and Estradiol-17β in Various Plasmas

Subjects or patients	Age (range)	No. of subjects	μg/100 ml.	
			Estrone	Estradiol-17β
Normal women	18–33	4	0.015 (0.008–0.028)	0.031 (0.013–0.056)
Normal women			0.106 mid-cycle	0.023
			0.024 (day of end of menstrual flow)	0.009
Normal men	22–28	5	0.023 (0.010–0.036)	0.003 (<0.002–0.006)
Pregnancy 7th Month		1	1.03	0.55
9th Month		1	0.57	0.98
Granulosa cell tumor	30	1	0.33–0.37	0.18–0.19
Adrenal adenoma			0.128	0.076
Hirsutism Polycystic ovaries		7	0.070 (0.004–0.134)	0.021 (0.015–0.044)
Steer adrenal vein plasma (lyophilized)		2	0.100	0.028
			0.020	0.032
Women with ovarian dermoid cyst			0.998	0.085
Adrenal adenoma			0.035 before surgery	0.012
			0.005 after surgery	0.004

estrone and estradiol-17β titers in the plasma of normal women by a double isotope method employing S^{35} and I^{131}. These investigators found slightly more estradiol-17β than estrone and the mean of five samples was 0.024 μg of estrone and 0.037 μg of estradiol-17β. On a preliminary basis there appears to be a reasonable correspondence between the two methods.

The expected increases in both estrogens were found in the two pregnancy samples and on two samples from a patient who had a granulosa cell tumor.

Steer adrenal vein plasma from two different animals indicated estrone at the levels of 0.100 and 0.020 μg, and estradiol-17β was present at the 0.028 and 0.032 μg levels.

Two adrenal adenoma patients were studied, one with an elevated value for the estrogens and a second with normal values. The one patient with values in the normal range showed a drop from 0.035 to 0.005 μg per 100 ml plasma for estrone and a decrease from 0.012 to 0.004 μg for estradiol-17β after removal of the adenoma.

Seven subjects with hirsutism due to polycystic ovaries had a mean estradiol-17β concentration of 0.021 μg per 100 ml of plasma (range 0.015-0.044) which did not seem to vary significantly from that found for the limited observations for normal women, but the estrone value of 0.070 μg per 100 ml plasma for the hirsute women appeared to be significantly higher than that for normal women.

SUMMARY

The bulk, if not all, of estrogen biosynthesis proceeds through a route involving grossly acetate → cholesterol → androgen → estrogen. If testosterone is the example of the androgen, then the following pathways are indicated: testosterone → 19-hydroxytestosterone → estradiol-17β + formaldehyde; 19 hydroxytestosterone → 19-oxotestosterone → estradiol-17β + formic acid; 19 oxotestosterone → 10-carboxy-19-nortestosterone → 19-nortestosterone → estradiol-17β.

Estrone and estradiol-17β may be determined with a sensitivity of 0.002 μg using a combination of paper chromatographic, phosphoric acid fluorescence, and radioisotopic labeled estrogens for recovery correction. The same sensitivity may be attained using a double isotope method. The estrone and estradiol-17β concentration of plasma of normal menstruating women was 0.015 μg (0.008-0.028) and 0.031 μg (0.013-0.056) per 100 ml, while the concentration of these steroids in men's plasma was 0.023 μg (0.010-0.036) and 0.003 μg (<0.002-0.006) per 100 ml, respectively.

REFERENCES

1. Baggett, B., Engel, L. L., Savard, K., and Dorfman, R.I. 1955. *Federation Proc.* 14: 175.
2. Baggett, B., Engel, L. L., Savard, K., and Dorfman, R. I. 1956. *J. Biol. Chem.* 221: 931.
3. Dorfman, R. I., and Hamilton, J. B. 1939. *Endocrinology* 25: 33.
4. Gual, C., Morato, T., Hayano, M., Gut, M., and Dorfman, R.I. 1962. *Endocrinology* 71: 920.
5. Heard, R. D. H., Jellinck, P. H., and O'Donnell, V. J. 1955. *Endocrinology* 25: 33.
6. Heard, R. D. H., Jacobs, R., O'Donnell, V. J., Peron, F. J., Safran, J. C., Solomon, S. S., Thompson, L. M., Willoughby, H., and Yates, C. H. 1954A. *Recent Progr. Hormone Res.* 9: 383.
7. Heard, R. D. H., Jellinck, P. H., and O'Donnell, V. J. 1954. *Endocrinology* 54: 209.
8. Ichii, S., Forchielli, E., Perloff, W. H., and Dorfman, R. I. 1962. *Anal. Biochem.* 5: 422.
9. Longchampt, J. E., Gual, C., Ehrenstein, M., and Dorfman, R. I. 1960. *Endocrinology* 66: 416.
10. Meyer, A. S. 1955. *Experentia* 11: 99.
11. Meyer, A. S. 1955. *Biochim. Biophys. Acta* 17: 441.
12. Morato, T., Hayano, M., Dorfman, R. I., and Axelrod, L. R. 1961. *Biochem. Biophys. Res. Comm.* 6: 334.
13. Nathanson, J. T., and Towne, L. E. 1937. *Endocrinology* 25: 488.
14. Preedy, J. R. K. 1962. In *Methods in Hormone Research* (R. I. Dorfman, ed.), 1: 1, Academic Press, New York.
15. Ryan, K. J. 1959. *J. Biol. Chem.* 234: 268.
16. Steinach, E., and Kun, H. 1937. *Lancet* 2: 845.
17. Svendsen, R. 1960. *Acta Endocrinol.* 35: 161.
18. Werbin, H., Plotz, J., LeRoy, G. V., and Davis, M. E. 1957. *J. Am. Chem. Soc.* 79: 1012.
19. Wotiz, H. H., Davis, J. W., Lemon, H. M., and Gut, M. 1956. *J. Biol. Chem.* 222: 487.
20. Zondek, B. 1934. *Nature* 133: 494.

II

Ralph I. Dorfman, Ph.D.

BIOSYNTHESIS AND DETECTION OF ANDROGENS

This chapter, which deals with the biosynthesis of androgens and the determination of testosterone in plasma, will be particularly important to discussions of the hyperactive state of the ovaries discussed in Chapter 4.

ANDROGEN BIOSYNTHESIS

Six distinct pathways for the biosynthesis of androgens have been established or indicated. The mechanism, which has been described for all steroid-producing tissues and first reported by Slaunwhite and Samuels [20] and soon thereafter by Savard, et al. [21] involves the 17α-hydroxylation of progesterone, the formation of androst-4-ene-3, 17-dione by a desmolase reaction, and the reduction of the 17-keto group to testosterone (Fig. 2-1). This path is known for the testis, [20], [21], for the ovaries [22], [12], and in the adrenals [18].

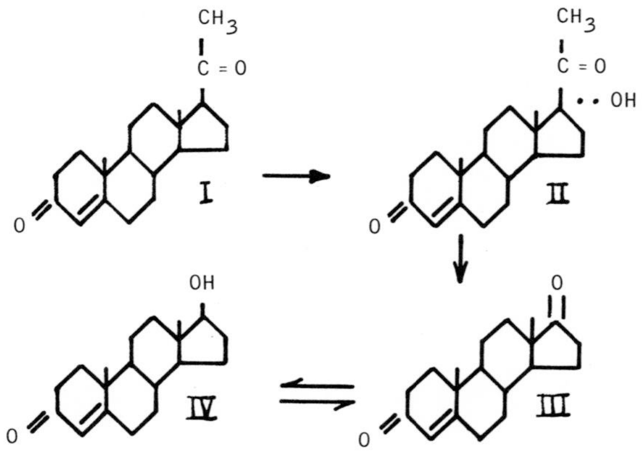

Fig. 2-1. Biosynthesis Androgens

I.   Progesterone
II. 17α-Hydroxy-progesterone
III. Androst-4-ene-3,17-dione
IV. Testosterone

Evidence for the second pathway (Fig. 2-2) involving the formation of dehydroepiandrosterone rests on secure grounds. Incubations of a homogenate prepared from a human adrenal adenoma with pregnenolone-7-H^3 resulted in the formation of dehydroepiandrosterone-H^3 [10]. The same conversion was reported by Burstein and Dorfman [1], who injected the tritium-labeled substrate into a virilized woman bearing an adrenal adenoma and isolated tritiated dehydroepiandrosterone from her urine in good yield. The step 17α-hydroxypregnenolone to dehydroepiandrosterone has been established by Solomon, et al. [23]. The isolation of dehydroepiandrosterone from testis by Neher and Wettstein [14] disproved the thesis that this androgen is exclusively of adrenal origin.

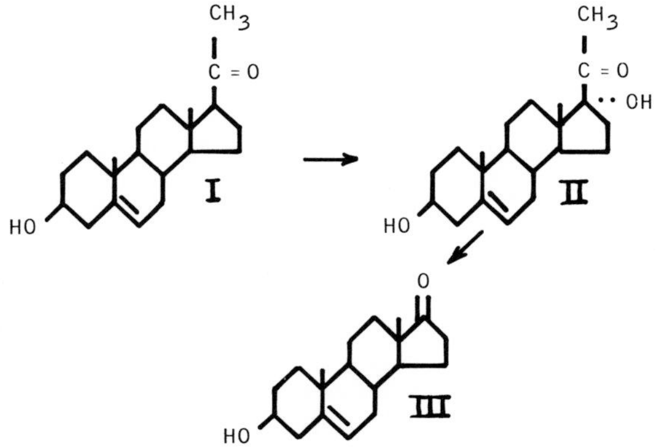

Fig. 2-2. Biosynthesis of Androgens

I. Pregnenolone
II. 17α-Hydroxypregnenolone
III. Dehydroepiandrosterone

The third pathway for androgen biosynthesis (Fig. 2-3), involving the conversion of progesterone to testosterone acetate and finally to testosterone, is indicated from the studies of Kase, et al. [13], who found that the incubation of progesterone-7-H^3 and 17α-hydroxyprogesterone-4-C^{14}, with a homogenate prepared from human polycystic ovaries, yielded testosterone containing a higher ratio of H^3/C^{14} than that found for androst-4-ene-3,17-dione simultaneously formed. This suggests the possibility that testosterone could be formed from progesterone without the prior formation of androst-4-ene-3,17-dione. This mechanism has been established by Fonken, et al. [6], who isolated the necessary testosterone acetate intermediate in the transformation of progesterone to testosterone by *Cladosporium resinae*. It is possible that this direct pathway is important in supplying highly active testosterone from normal testes and abnormal ovaries and adrenals in hirsute or virilized women.

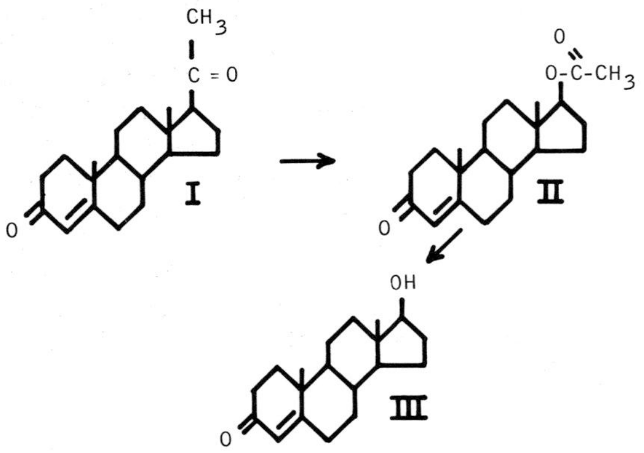

Fig. 2-3.   Biosynthesis of Androgens

I.   Progesterone
II.   Testosterone Acetate
III.   Testosterone

A possible fourth mechanism is the direct formation of dehydro-epiandrosterone from cholesterol without the necessity of a C_{21} inter-mediate. It is visualized that $17\alpha,20\alpha$-dihydroxycholesterol may be the intermediate. This is a reasonable possibility on the basis of *in vivo* [1] and *in vitro* studies [11](Fig. 2-4).

The bulk of dehydroepiandrosterone is secreted as the sulfate and even if secreted into the blood as the free compound it would be rapidly converted to the conjugate. As the conjugate this androgen may be considered to be relatively inert. However, recent unpublished studies have indicated that the intravenous administration of tritiated dehydro-epiandrosterone resulted in the appearance of testosterone-H^3 and androst-4-ene-3,17-dione-H^3 in the blood. This transformation oc-curs in men in the absence of the testis and in women in the absence of the ovary. Proof is not absolute that the reactions take place solely in the adrenal and it is quite likely that this biosynthetic route to tes-tosterone and androst-4-ene-3,17-dione (Fig. 2-5) may take place in the gonads and adrenals, and in peripheral tissues.

The sixth and final pathway is related to peripheral formation of androgens from nonandrogenic compounds by enzymes in such tissues as liver and muscle. Oertel and Eik-Nes [16] have suggested that dehydroepiandrosterone may be formed from pregnenolone and 17α-hydroxypregnenolone by striated muscle tissue.

The formation of C_{19} from C_{21} steroids with liver preparations is well documented. C_{21}-compounds having oxygen functions at C-17 and C-20 are metabolized to 17-ketosteroids [4]. Typical examples are given in Fig. 2-6. Many *in vivo* experiments have been reported using the following substrates: cortisone, cortisol, 21-deoxycortisone,

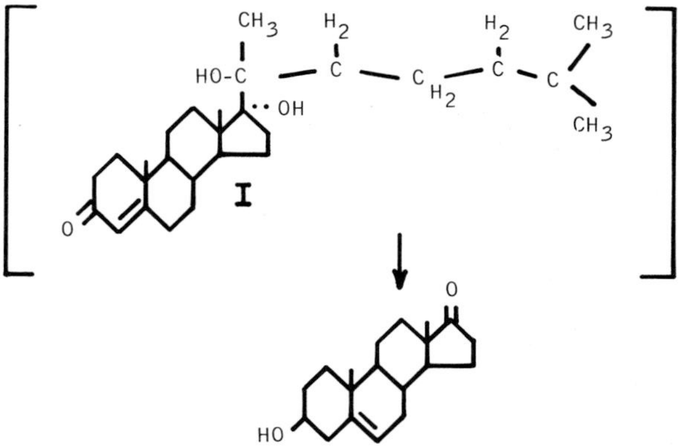

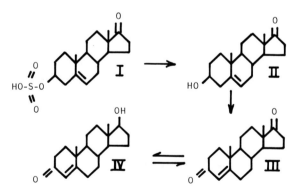

Fig. 2-4. Biosynthesis of Androgens

    I. 17α,20α-Dihydrocholesterol (not isolated)
   II. Dehydroepiandrosterone

21-deoxycortisol, 11-deoxycortisol, and 17α-hydroxyprogesterone.
The yield of 17-ketosteroids from C_{21} steroids possessing the Δ^5-3β-
hydroxyl groups is severely reduced. *In vitro* methods have been
quite illuminating, such as those of Caspi and Hechter [2], [3],
Forchielli and Dorfman [8] and Forchielli, et al. [9], where 11-
deoxycortisol incubated with liver homogenates has yielded androsterone, androstane-3,17-dione, Δ^4-androstene-3,17-dione, and
etiocholanolene. The cellular location of the desmolase has not been
established.

Fig. 2-5. Biosynthesis of Androgens

    I. Dehydroepiandrosterone Sulfate
   II. Dehydroepiandrosterone
  III. Androst-4-ene-3,17-dione
  IV. Testosterone

Androgen biosynthetic pathways already discussed do not include the route to 11-oxygenated androgens. The two important members of this group, andrenosterone and 11β-hydroxyandrost-4-ene, 17-dione, are interconvertible; they are produced by two routes: by 11β-hydroxylation of androst-4-ene-3, 17-dione and by conversion from C_{21} steroids such as cortisol and/or 11-deoxycortisol.

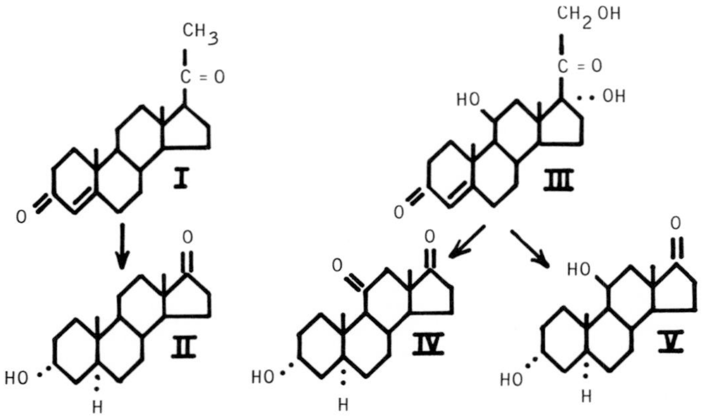

Fig. 2-6. Biosynthesis of Androgens

    I. 17α-Hydroxyprogesterone
   II.   Androsterone
  III.   Cortisol
  IV.   11-Ketoandrosterone
   V. 11β-Hydroxyandrosterone

BLOOD ANDROGENS

All too often patients with frank hirsutism and/or virilism have little or no changes in their titer of urinary and/or blood 17-ketosteroids. This is due apparently to a relatively high daily production of relatively inactive androgens such as dehydroepiandrosterone and androst-4-ene-3, 17-dione which are responsible for the bulk of the 17-ketosteroids. In the normal woman a daily production of 18 mg of these compounds in fact yields about 9 mg of urinary 17-ketosteroids, and about 2 mg of testosterone would yield about 1 mg of urinary 17-ketosteroids. Even if the level of daily testosterone production would increase by 100 per cent to 4 mg the net increase in total 17-ketosteroids would be only 1 mg and hardly important although the biological stimulation could be highly significant.

A number of ways could be suggested to improve our methods of evaluating the abnormal androgenic state due to either hyperactivity or hypoactivity. One way might be to use the testosterone secretion or production rate if it is assumed that the amount of active hormone available at the target site is a function of the secretion rate. A second improved method might be the evaluation of the level of free testosterone in blood, assuming that this value is related to the concentration of the active component at the target site.

Both methods have been developed with the plasma testosterone methods furnishing considerably more data at the present time.

In a preliminary report, Finkelstein, et al. [7] described a method for the estimation of free testosterone in the peripheral plasma from normal men and women. Plasma from men and virilized females contained significantly more testosterone than plasma obtained from normal women. Since the appearance of this preliminary communication, Oertel [15] has reported on a method for measuring testosterone levels in plasma, and Oertel and Kaiser [17] have measured levels of this androgen in the plasma of young male subjects. At the Worcester Foundation, the method has been improved and testosterone plasma values have been obtained in a larger series of normal men and women, hirsute and virilized women. The influence of ovariectomy, adrenalectomy, wedge resection, prednisone, and human chorionic gonadotropin on plasma testosterone has also been studied.

A TESTOSTERONE METHOD [5, 7]

The plasma was prepared from freshly drawn blood by centrifugation. Either citrate solution or heparin may be used as the anticoagulant. Plasma so prepared may be stored in the frozen state up to six months. For the analysis, the plasma was divided into two equal portions, A and B. A tracer quantity of testosterone-C^{14} (about 2000 cpm and weighing less than 0.02 μg) which would serve as an internal recovery control was added to Portion A. Portion B served as the plasma blank and this was treated identically to A in all respects except that it was not incubated with the placental enzyme. Alcohol was added prior to the addition of the enzyme preparation and cofactors to denature the enzymes and inhibit any possible side reactions. The extraction and treatment of the plasma extract and isolation of the testosterone zone by paper chromatography was identical to that previously reported [7].

A microsomal pellet containing the aromatizing enzyme system was prepared from human term placenta, according to Ryan [19], resuspended in water, lyophilized, and the dried powder stored in a dessiccator at -10 degrees. Five-tenths of 1 mg of this dried powder converts 1-2 μg of testosterone quantitatively to estrogenic material. This represents better than a twenty-fold reduction in the weight of the enzyme preparation compared to the preparation previously described [7].

The eluate of the testosterone zone obtained from the paper chromatogram was concentrated to a small volume, transferred to 10 ml beakers, and evaporated to dryness. To this residue there was added 1.0 mg of the placental enzyme suspended in 0.5 ml of 0.1 M phosphate buffer at pH 7.0, 5 μMoles of glucose-6-phosphate, 100 μg TPH, and 0.1 Kornberg unit of glucose-6-phosphate dehydrogenase in 0.5 ml 0.154 M KCL. The mixture was incubated for one hour at 37 degrees in air.

The reaction was stopped by the addition of 5.0 ml of absolute ethanol and the insoluble material separated by centrifugation. The precipitate and residue remaining in the beaker was washed two times with 5 ml portions of absolute ethanol followed by centrifugation each time. The combined alcoholic supernatant solutions were treated with 2-4 mg of sodium borohydride and allowed to stand at room temperature for 15 minutes. This step was introduced to reduce any estrone present to estradiol-17β, thus yielding a single uniform end product. The reaction mixture was concentrated to a small volume (1.0 ml) in a stream of nitrogen and diluted to 10 ml with water. After the addition of two to three drops of 1 N acetic acid (to neutralize any alkali formed from the decomposition of the borohydride) the mixture was extracted with 3-10 ml portions of fresh distilled benzene. The combined benzene extracts were washed with a small volume of water, dried over sodium sulfate, and concentrated to dryness. A partition into phenolic and neutral fractions was considered unnecessary since the small amounts of neutral material remaining after the enzyme reaction could be readily separated from the estradiol-17β by paper chromatography.

The chromatography and estimation of estradiol-17β were carried out as previously described [7]. The number of C^{14} counts obtained in the estradiol-17β served as the index of recovery and all values were corrected for losses on this basis.

Using this method [5], plasma testosterone values have been obtained on various subjects (Table 2-1). The influence of various surgical procedures and treatments on plasma testosterone levels have also been reported (Table 2-2). Nine men varying in age from 23 to 74 years had plasma testosterone values varying from 0.1 to 0.98 μg per 100 ml and a mean value of 0.56 μg. The corresponding plasma testosterone values obtained on ten normal women, 23 to 35 years of age, ranged from 0.02 to 0.26. Each of the subjects had a normal cycle and was not hirsute (Table 2-1). The same table presents the plasma levels of two groups of hirsute women. One group had proved polycystic ovaries and was classed as having the Stein-Leventhal syndrome. The mean 17-ketosteroid value for this group of six women, ranging in age from 18 to 41 years, was 12.2 (7-24) mg per twenty-four hours. The blood testosterone values ranged from 0.25 to 0.42 μg/100 ml with a mean of 0.33 μg per 100 ml. The second group of four women was hirsute, but the diagnosis was not established. The mean testosterone value for this group was 0.25 μg (0.11 to 0.32 μg) per 100 ml plasma, and the mean 17-ketosteroid values were 13.7 mg/day.

Table 2-1. Testosterone in Human Plasma (Data of Forchielli, et al. [5])

Subjects (age range)	No.	17-Ketosteroids mg per day	Mean testosterone µg/100 ml (range)
Normal men (23-74)	9	-	0.56 (0.1-0.98)
Normal women (22-35)	10	-	0.12 (0.02-0.26)
Hirsute women		12.2	0.33
Polycystic ovaries (Stein-Leventhal type) (18-41)	6	(7-24)	(0.25-0.42)
Hirsute women (Diagnosis not established) (14-47)	4	13.7 (8-18)	0.25 (0.11-0.32)
Virilized women Polycystic ovaries (Stein-Leventhal type) (14-36)	5	10.9 (6.4-20)	0.49 (0.30-0.74)
Ovarian hilus cell tumor (68)	1	2-4	2.0* before surgery 0.02 after 0.05 surgery 0.04
Women with adrenal adenoma	4	1000	1.3*
		250-1000	1.4
		308	0.22 before surgery
			0.02 after surgery
		200-272	0.79†

*These values were published previously (Finkelstein, et al., [7])
†Also bilateral polycystic ovaries

Five subjects had the stigma of virilization, and the blood testosterone values were considerably elevated. The mean value of 0.49 μg per 100 ml of plasma was quite similar to that found for the normal men. Of particular interest is the fact that the 17-ketosteroid mean value for this group was only 10.9 mg per day. Only one patient had an elevated 17-ketosteroid titer of 20 mg.

Plasma testosterone levels were studied in four women bearing virilizing adrenal adenomas. All had greatly elevated 17-ketosteroids and three of the patients had very high testosterone levels. One subject had a value of 0.22 μg per 100 ml, which was in the normal range, which decreased to 0.02 μg after the tumor was removed. Of further interest was the relative lack of virilism but severe hirsutism in this subject.

The presurgical value of 2 μg/100 ml plasma for the patient with a hilus cell tumor had been reported previously. After surgery the plasma level of testosterone dropped considerably to 0.02, 0.04, 0.05 μg/100 ml.

Ovariectomy of hirsute women produced a decrease in blood testosterone; the extent, however, varied from subject to subject. In one virilized Stein-Leventhal patient who had the excessive plasma testosterone level of 0.71 μg bilateral ovariectomy decreased this value to 0.22 μg per 100 ml. The mean value for all five ovariectomized women was 0.11 μg and no different from the mean plasma testosterone value of 0.12 for the normal women. This may be an indication that at least some of the patients had elevated testosterone because of hyperfunctioning testosterone biosynthetic mechanisms other than the ovary. Extra-ovarian sources of testosterone were also indicated in the patient who had been bilaterally adrenalectomized.

Decreases in plasma testosterone were effected by wedge resection and by prednisolone treatment (Table 2-2). The surgical procedure caused a net decrease of 0.41 μg per 100 ml of plasma from a mean of 0.63 μg to 0.22 μg. Prednisolone effected a change from 0.34 μg to 0.07, indicating a net decrease of 0.27 μg of plasma testosterone.

In one hirsute ovariectomized patient not listed in Table 2-2, the plasma testosterone of 0.15 μg was decreased to 0.05 μg when the patient was treated daily with 8 mg of 6α-methyl-prednisolone plus 3000 I.U. of chorionic gonadotropin (Follutein, Squibb and Co.). This resulted in a plasma testosterone level of 0.01, indicating no significant change. This experiment is of particular interest since it illustrates quite clearly the relation directly or indirectly of the adrenal to testosterone formation.

The adrenalectomized subject (Table 2-2) was treated once daily for three days with 3000 I.U. of human chorionic gonadotropin. The change of 0.08 μg per 100 ml plasma to 0.09 μg per 100 ml plasma as a result of this stimulation was not significant, but stimulation of plasma estrogens was definite. The pretreatment levels of estrone of

0.020 μg increased to 0.080 μg while the estradiol-17β level rose from <0.002 to 0.016 μg.

Table 2-2

Influence of Surgery and Treatment on Testosterone in Plasma [5]

Subjects (no.)	Treatment	Mean testosterone μg/100 ml	
Hirsute women (5)	Ovariectomy	0.11 (0.04-0.22)	
Bilaterally adrenalectomized women	25 mg Cortisone plus 1 mg Fluoxymestrone daily	0.08 0.09	(During treatment with 3000 I.U. human chorionic gonado- tropin)
Hirsute women (3)	Wedge resection	Before 0.53 0.77 0.58	After 0.11 0.34 0.22
Hirsute women (4)	Prednisone treatment 10-20 mg/day	Before 0.48 0.44 0.1 -	After 0.13 0.07 0.02 0.16

SUMMARY

Six biosynthetic pathways have been established or indicated for androgen formation. These include (1) progesterone → 17α-hydroxy-progesterone, androst-4-ene-3,17-dione → testosterone; (2) pregnen-olone → 17α-hydroxypregnenolone → dehydroepiandrosterone; (3) pro-gesterone → testosterone acetate → testosterone; (4) cholesterol → 17α, 20α-dihydroxycholesterol → dehydroepiandrosterone → androst-4-ene-3,17-dione → testosterone; (6) C_{21} to C_{19} steroids. To supplement these biosynthetic reactions, C_{19} steroids such as androst-4-ene-3,17-dione may be hydroxylated in the adrenal at carbon 11 forming 11β-hydroxy-androst-4-ene-3,17-dione.

The importance of secretion rates and/or concentration plasma of testosterone is discussed. A method is described for estimated plas-ma testosterone levels and typical results are recorded for normal men and women as well as hirsute, virilized, adrenalectomized, and gonadectomized subjects. Plasma testosterone levels are elevated in hirsute and virilized women and decreased by ovariectomy and by adrenalectomy. Cortical treatment and wedge resection also decrease plasma testosterone levels.

REFERENCES

1. Burstein, S., and Dorfman, R. I. 1962. *Acta Endocrinol.* **40**: 188.
2. Caspi, E., and Hechter, O. 1954. *Arch. Biochem. Biophys.* **52**: 478.
3. Caspi, E., and Hechter, O. 1956. *Arch. Biochem. Biophys.* **61**: 299.
4. Dorfman, R. I. 1957. *Ann. Rev. Biochem.* **26**: 523.
5. Forchielli, E., Sorchini, G., Nightingale, M., Brust, N., and Dorfman, R. I. 1963. *Anal. Biochem.* **5**: 416.
6. Fonken, G. S., Murray, H. C., and Reineke, L. M. 1960. *J. Am. Chem. Soc.* **82**: 5507.
7. Finkelstein, M., Forchielli, E., and Dorfman, R. I. 1961. *J. Clin. Endocrinol. & Metab.* **21**: 98.
8. Forchielli, E., and Dorfman, R. I. 1956. *J. Biol Chem.* **223**: 443.
9. Forchielli, E., Rosenkrantz, H., and Dorfman, R. I. 1955. *J. Biol. Chem.* **215**: 713.
10. Goldstein, M., Gut, M., and Dorfman, R. I. 1960. *Biochim. Biophys. Acta* **38**: 190.
11. Gual, C., Lemus, A. E., Kline, I. T., Gut, M., and Dorfman, R. I. 1962. *J. Clin. Endocrinol. & Metab.* **22**: 1193.
12. Kase, N., Forchielli, E., and Dorfman, R. I. 1961. *Acta Endocrinol.* **37**: 19.
13. Kase, N., Forchielli, E., and Dorfman, R. I. 1963. Unpublished.
14. Neher, R., and Wettstein, A. 1960. *Acta Endocrinol.* **35**: 1.
15. Oertel, G. W. 1961. *Acta Endocrinol.* **37**: 237.
16. Oertel, G. W., and Eik-Nes, K. B. 1959. *Endocrinology* **65**: 766.
17. Oertel, G. W., and Kaiser, H. E. 1961. *Klinishe Wchschr.* **39**: 1146.
18. Rao, B. G., and Heard, R. D. H. 1957. *Arch. Biochem. Biophys.* **66**: 504.
19. Ryan, K. J. 1959. *J. Biol. Chem.* **235**: 268.
20. Slaunwhite, W. R., Jr., and Samuels, L. T. 1956. *J. Biol. Chem.* **220**: 341.
21. Savard, K., Dorfman, R. I., Baggett, B., and Engel, L. L. 1956. *J. Clin. Endocrinol. & Metab.* **16**: 1629.
22. Solomon, S., van de Wiele, R., and Lieberman, S. 1956. *J. Am. Chem. Soc.* **78**: 5453.
23. Solomon, S., Carter, A. C., and Lieberman, S. 1960. *J. Biol. Chem.* **235**: 351.

III

Ralph I. Dorfman, Ph.D.
ESTIMATION OF "EFFECTIVE" STEROID HORMONE CONCENTRATIONS

For the many years since the discovery of biologically active steroids, efforts have been made to quantitate these compounds in body fluids. Such studies were necessary for the elucidation of fundamental problems in biology and for practical clinical studies. An approach to this general problem will be considered in this chapter and is modeled after a previous publication dealing primarily with the hormones of the adrenal cortex [3].

Specifically, this chapter will consider the active steroids in blood, define the concept of unique metabolites, discuss the unique metabolites of the known active steroids and the biosynthetic intermediates. The latter compounds are particularly important in genetic-hormonal defects since biosynthetic blocks, partial or complete, result in excessive concentrations of intermediates which in turn give rise to corresponding urinary catabolites. It is obvious that good analyses of these catabolites can lead to more exact knowledge of the genetic defect.

BIOLOGICALLY ACTIVE STEROIDS IN BLOOD PLASMA

A biologically active steroid is one which is carried in an easily available form in the blood. Although this appears to be a reasonable hypothesis, the question may be asked whether analyses for these components can be done with presently available methods. The answer is basically yes with the promise that the method either has been developed or can be developed utilizing presently available methods.

Fig. 3-1 details the thirteen biologically active steroids which may play significant physiological roles normally and, when the plasma concentration is modified, cause significant pathology. The components progesterone, aldosterone, and cortisol need no further comments. Deoxycorticosterone is a minor component when one considers electrolyte control, but in the congenital adrenal hyperplasia syndrome when the 11β-hydroxylase variant is considered, the concentration of deoxycorticosterone may increase considerably; thus its increment in blood actually becomes of some importance.

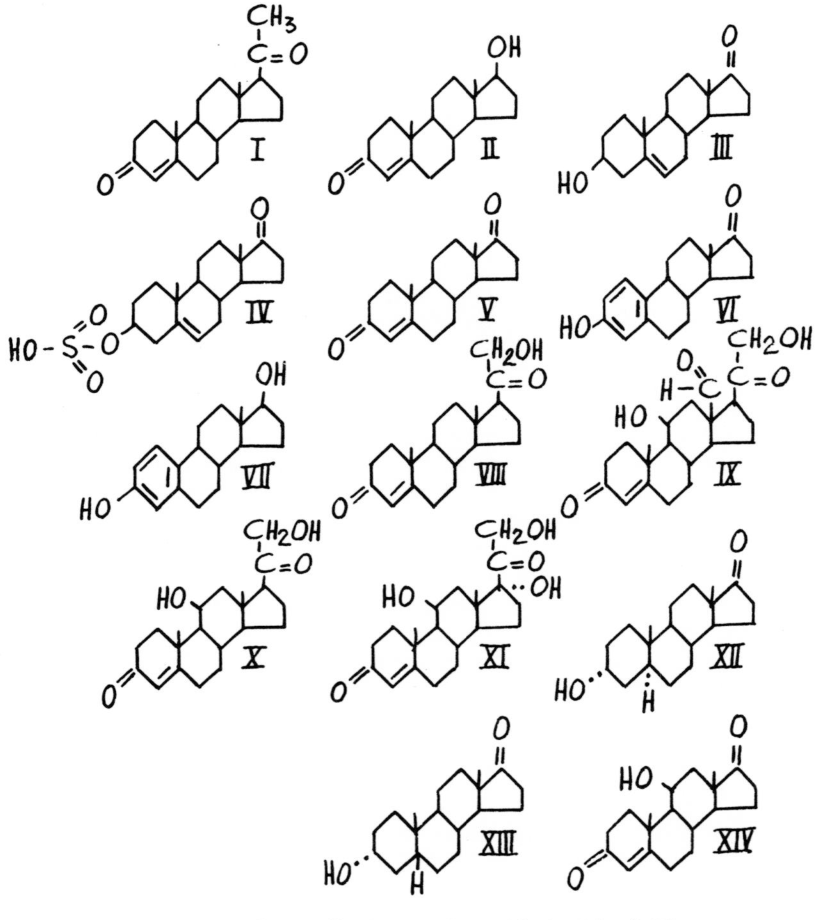

Fig. 3-1. Biologically Active Steroids in Blood Plasma

I.	Progesterone	VIII.	Deoxycorticosterone
II.	Testosterone	IX.	Aldosterone
III.	Dehydroepiandrosterone	X.	Corticosterone
IV.	Dehydroepiandrosterone sulfate	XI.	Cortisol
V.	Androst-4-ene-3,17-dione	XII.	Androsterone
VI.	Estrone	XIII.	Etiocholanolone
VII.	Estradiol-17β	XIV.	11β-Hydroxyandrost-4-ene-3,17-dione

The concentration of estrogens in plasma, when viewed from the classical estrogen viewpoint, may be considered to be the free estrone and estradiol-17β contents of plasma. Methods for the determination of these components and the arguments for such studies are presented in Chapter 1.

Still to be determined is the physiological meaning of the estrogen conjugates. Are these compounds active per se? This question cannot be answered at present.

The question of androgenicity and testosterone and other androgens has already been discussed in Chapter 2. There remains only the need to summarize the main points. Testosterone appears to be present as the free compound in plasma. Only about 10 per cent of the total is conjugated. The small proportion is present as both the glucuronide and sulfate. Free testosterone is generally the main androgen since it is some twenty or more times as active as dehydroepiandrosterone, the corresponding sulfate, or androst-4-ene-3, 17-dione. Progesterone is essentially *the* progestational hormone and this activity in plasma is only modified slightly by the presence of some 20_α- and 20_β-reduced compounds which have only limited activity. Corticoid activity in humans is represented by free cortisol; corticosterone is far less active, but blood determinations of this component could be of real value in certain states due to abnormal steroid biosynthesis.

The $C_{19}O_2$ metabolites are included in this list as steroids which exert a "nonclassical" type of activity. Etiocholanolone has been associated with a type of periodic fever, while androsterone is associated with blood cholesterol levels.

UNIQUE METABOLITES

The problem of the active steroid evaluation involves the determination of the steroid hormones and/or metabolites which are indicators of single components. Any metabolite which indicates one and only one tissue steroid is termed a unique metabolite.

The biosynthesis of pregnenolone from cholesterol involves at least three intermediates, as indicated in Fig. 3-2. The presence of these hydroxylated intermediates in plasma may be of diagnostic importance. At the present time they have not been identified in blood, and this identification is necessary before further speculation would be profitable. Steroid hormones and related substances need not be produced in one and only one gland. Many of the steroid hormones are produced in most of the steroid-producing tissues, and frequently a substance is produced predominantly in one gland rather than in that gland exclusively. Specific overlapping in production from gland to gland seriously interferes with evaluating the functional status of a single gland.

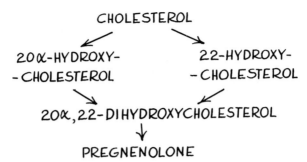

Fig. 3-2. Biosynthesis of Pregnenolone

The unique metabolites of the biologically important steroids are presented in Figs. 3-3 through 3-6. Pregnanediol is considered to be the principal and a unique metabolite of progesterone, and the catabolic reactions of this steroid in ring A are characteristic for the C_{21} class of steroids. The Δ^3-ketone in ring A for C_{21} steroids is reduced primarily to the $3\alpha, 5\beta$ configuration. The corresponding steroids in Fig. 3-3, deoxycorticosterone and 11β-hydroxyprogesterone, similarly are reduced primarily to the $3\alpha, 5\beta$ forms. Probably the unique metabolite of pregnenolone is the 20α-reduced form, Δ^5-pregnene-3β-20α-diol. Pregnenolone as such has not been detected in blood or urine.

Neither progesterone nor pregnenolone is produced exclusively in a single gland. Both steroids are important biosynthetic intermediates in the gonads and placenta and will, of course, complicate seriously any attempt for adrenal status evaluation in women during the luteal phase of the cycle as well as in pregnancy. The real utility of these indicators is in men or in ovariectomized women. Even studies in women during the follicular phase of the cycle may be confusing. Increased excretion of pregnanediol and/or pregn-5-ene-$3\beta, 20\alpha$-diol may arise from the ovary or adrenal or both.

Fig. 3-4 considers three additional C_{21}-Δ^4-3-ketones, 17α-hydroxyprogesterone, 21-deoxycortisol and corticosterone, all of which undergo ring A reduction during catabolism. 17α-hydroxyprogesterone, in addition to ring A reduction, is also reduced at carbon 20, forming pregnanetriol (pregnane-$3\alpha, 17\alpha, 20\alpha$-triol). The fourth compound, 17α-hydroxypregnenolone, is primarily reduced to the 20α-hydroxy derivative which is the unique metabolite. The Δ^5-3β-hydroxy configuration cannot arise from the Δ^4-3-ketone, so that pregn-5-ene-3β, $17\alpha, 20\alpha$-triol specifically represents endogenously produced 17α-hydroxypregnenolone.

Cortisol undergoes metabolic changes at carbon atoms 3, 4, 5, 11 and 20, as well as side chain removal, and the number of known catabolites has been set at eleven in a recent study. For practical purposes, however, the two tetrahydro derivatives urocortisol ($3\alpha, 11\beta, 17\alpha, 21$-tetrahydroxypregnan-20-one) and urocortisone

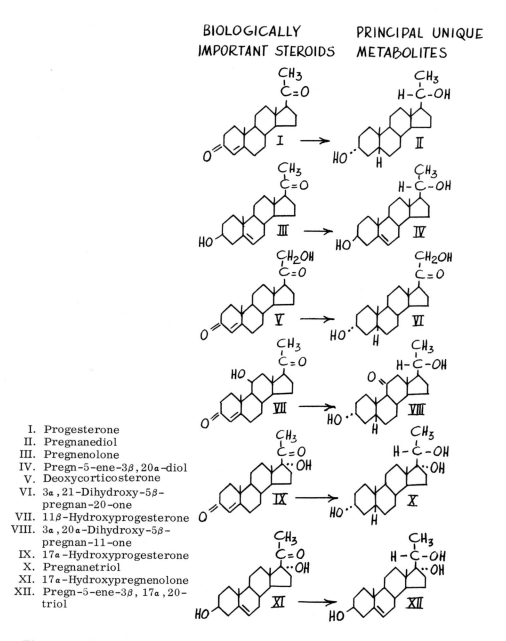

I. Progesterone
II. Pregnanediol
III. Pregnenolone
IV. Pregn-5-ene-3β,20α-diol
V. Deoxycorticosterone
VI. 3α,21-Dihydroxy-5β-
    pregnan-20-one
VII. 11β-Hydroxyprogesterone
VIII. 3α,20α-Dihydroxy-5β-
    pregnan-11-one
IX. 17α-Hydroxyprogesterone
X. Pregnanetriol
XI. 17α-Hydroxypregnenolone
XII. Pregn-5-ene-3β,17α,20-
    triol

Fig. 3-3. $C_{21}O_2$ and $C_{21}O_3$ Steroids and Their Principal Unique Catabolites

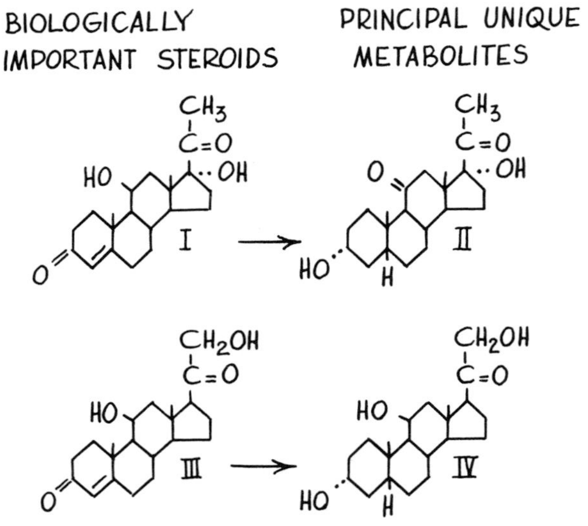

BIOLOGICALLY
IMPORTANT STEROIDS

PRINCIPAL UNIQUE
METABOLITES

Fig. 3-4. $C_{21}O_4$ Steroids and Their Principal Unique Catabolites

I. 21-Deoxycortisol
II. $3\alpha,17\alpha$-Dihydroxy-5β-pregnane-3, 20-dione

III. Corticosterone
IV. $3\alpha,11\beta,21$-Trihydroxy-5β-pregnan- 20-one

($3\alpha,17\alpha,21$-trihydroxypregnane-11,20-dione) may be considered unique metabolites (Fig. 3-5).

The evaluation of testosterone production cannot be accomplished by the analysis of either blood or urine for androsterone and etiocholanolone, since these latter steroids arise primarily from dehydroepiandrosterone and androst-4-ene-3,17-dione. The only possibility available at the present time is testosterone in blood (which was previously discussed), perhaps urine concentration as indicated by the report of Schubert [7], or possibly the concentration of 5α-androst-16-en-3α-ol in the urine (Fig. 3-6).

There seems to be growing evidence that 5α-androst-16-en-3α-ol is in fact a unique metabolite of testosterone, but reasonable certainty has not been approached. Cholesterol-4-C^{14} and pregnenolone-7α-H^{3}, when administered intraveneously to a woman suffering from a massive virilizing adrenal adenoma, did result in the excretion of excessive quantities of 5α-androst-16-en-3α-ol-C^{14}-H^{3} [2]. The incubation of testosterone with rat testis yielded two Δ^{16}-steroids, 5α-androst-16-en-3β-ol and androst-4,16-dien-3-one [9], and the latter compound was also realized when testosterone was incubated with human liver [10]. These studies demonstrate that Δ^{16}-steroids are in fact derived by usual biosynthetic pathways from cholesterol and that a direct relation between Δ^{16} steroids and testosterone has been established. It is unlikely that Δ^{16} compounds can be derived from 17-ketosteroids such as androst-4-ene-3,17-dione and dehydroepiandrosterone, but the possibility of the conversion of androstane-3α,17α-diol to 5α-androst-16-en-3α-ol requires investigation.

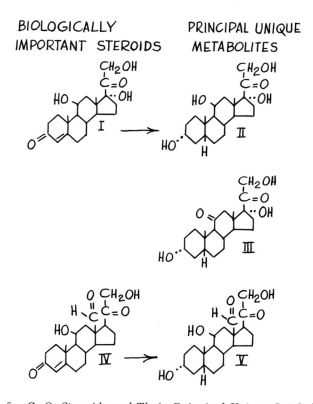

Fig. 3-5. $C_{21}O_5$ Steroids and Their Principal Unique Catabolites

I. Cortisol   IV. Aldosterone
II. Urocortisol   V. Uroaldosterone
III. Urocortisone

The fact that incubation of testosterone with rat testis yielded the 3β- rather than the 3α-Δ^{16}-stereoisomer is not particularly troublesome since this may be due to species difference, or it may be that both the 3 - and 3β-steroids were produced but that the former form was present in too low a concentration to be detected. Boar testis contains 5α-androst-16-en-3α-ol and 5α-androst-16-en-3β-ol [6].

It is of interest that the urinary concentration of 5α-androst-16-en-3α-ol is increased in the urines of virilized women. The increase has been found whether the abnormality involved the adrenal or the ovary. Preliminary studies by Brooksbank and Haslewood have indicated the possibility that the concentration of the Δ^{16}-compound is higher in the urine of men than of women, but variations have been exceedingly great. Additional studies are needed to establish this point with any reasonable certainty.

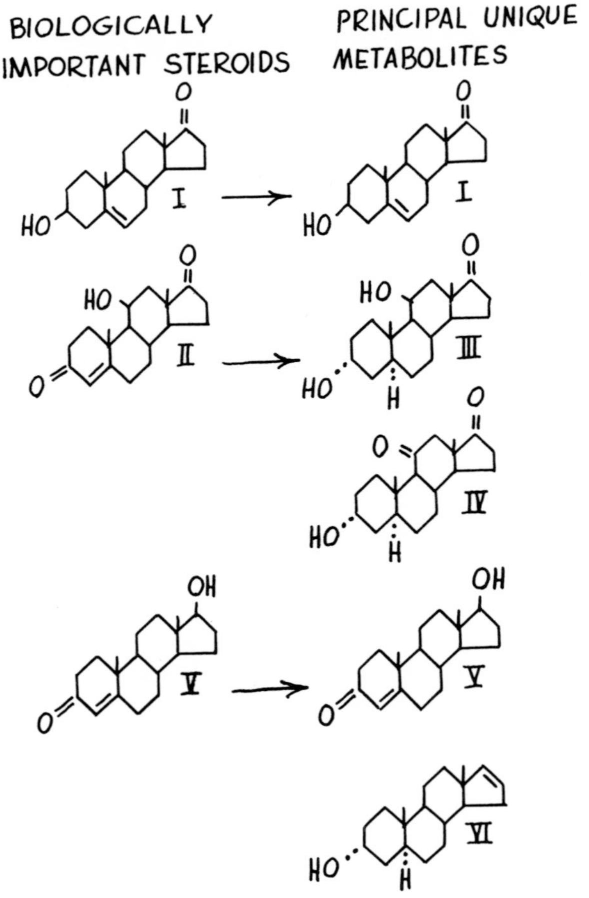

Fig. 3-6. $C_{19}O_2$ Steroids and Their Principal Unique Catabolites

I. Dehydroepiandrosterone
II. 11β-Hydroxyandrost-3-ene-3,17-dione
III. 11β-Hydroxyandrosterone
IV. 11-Ketoandrosterone
V. Testosterone
VI. 5α-Androst-16-en-3α-ol

At the present time the best indicator of testosterone production is the blood concentration of this steroid, but even this measure is not without difficulties. Some testosterone circulating in blood may arise

from androst-4-ene-3, 17-dione secreted into the blood or Δ^4-andro-
stene-3, 17-dione originating from secreted dehydroepiandrosterone.
A second complicating factor is the possibility of the formation in the
adrenal and secretion into the blood of androst-5-ene-3β, 17β-diol.
This steroid on ring A oxidation would yield testosterone. Thus testosterone in blood is perhaps a better measure of the androgenic stim-
ulus than a precise indicator of the exact quantities of testosterone
produced as such in the gland.

The question of unique metabolites of dehydroepiandrosterone has
not been adequately resolved. The measure of blood and urinary dehydroepiandrosterone appears to be a reasonable approach. Fortunately
no appreciable quantity of dehydroepiandrosterone is formed periph-
erally from Δ^4-3-keto steroids. Thus androst-4-ene-3, 17-dione, for
all practical purposes, is not converted to dehydroepiandrosterone.
Complications do arise with respect to androst-5-ene-3β, 17β-diol,
which is an adrenal product but at a concentration less than 1 per cent
of that of the dehydroepiandrosterone secreted [4]. This steroid on
oxidation at carbon 17 will obviously yield dehydroepiandrosterone.

Recent studies by Baulieu [1] have shown that although an adrenal
virilizing tumor contained no free dehydroepiandrosterone, this steroid was present in relatively high concentration as the sulfate. Further,
in the same patient, the adrenal venous blood contained no free dehydroepiandrosterone but an exceedingly high amount of the sulfate was present. The concentration of free dehydroepiandrosterone in adrenal
venous blood is distinctly lower than that of peripheral blood. Even
after stimulation with ACTH [8], free dehydroepiandrosterone in adrenal venous blood was lower than found in peripheral blood.

Until recently it was believed that dehydroepiandrosterone was
produced exclusively by the adrenal. This view must now be altered,
since Neher and Wettstein [5] have isolated dehydroepiandrosterone
from testis tissue, and these investigators have also shown that pregnenolone and 17α-hydroxypregnenolone may be converted to dehydroepiandrosterone by testis tissue. It is still possible that under normal conditions the dehydroepiandrosterone contribution by the adrenal
is so great as to make the testicular secretion negligible. Under abnormal conditions testicular and ovarian sources may be of considerable importance.

Consideration of the metabolism of androst-4-ene-3, 17-dione
brings up some difficult problems. First it must be noted that this
androgen is produced by all steroid-producing tissues, but it is likely
that under normal conditions the greatest amount of this steroid comes
from the adrenal gland. In women this is unquestionably true, but in
men the testis may normally contribute significant quantities. Of even
greater difficulty is the fact that androst-4-ene-3, 17-dione in circulation may arise from testosterone, dehydroepiandrosterone and androst-
5-ene-3β, 17β-diol and that these three compounds as well as androst-
4-ene-3, 17-dione all are metabolized to androsterone and etiocholanolone.

The two 11-oxygenated C_{19} steroids, 11β-hydroxyandrosterone and 11-ketoandrosterone, are the principal unique metabolites of 11β-hydroxy-androst-4-ene-3,17-dione (Fig. 3-6). Although there is some conversion of cortisol and cortisone to these $C_{21}O_3$ ring A reduced steroids, the amounts are minor and may be disregarded. When the quantity of cortisol and/or cortisone is severely increased, the additional amount of 11-oxygenated etiocholanolone derivatives are increased so greatly that the endogenous change can be easily recognized. No significant interference can be expected from the gonads, since no important quantity of 11β-hydroxy-androst-4-ene-3,17-dione is produced by these glands under normal conditions. Adrenosterone is unquestionably a secondary product derived from the 11β-hydroxy steroid and is also known to be metabolized primarily to the 5α-reduced 11-oxygenated 17-ketosteroids.

REFERENCES

1. Baulieu, E. E. 1960. *Compt. rend.* 248: 1421.
2. Burstein, S., and Dorfman, R. I. 1962. *Acta Endocrinol.* **40:** 188.
3. Dorfman, R. I. 1961. *Metabolism* 10: 902.
4. Hirschmann, H., DeCourcy, C., Levy, R. P., and Miller, K. L. 1960. *J. Biol. Chem.* 235: PC48.
5. Neher, R., and Wettstein, A. 1960. *Acta Endocrinol.* 35: 1.
6. Prelog, V., and Ruzicka, L. 1944. *Helv. chim. Acta.* 27: 61.
7. Schubert, K., and Wehrberger, K. 1960. *Naturwissenshaften* 47: 281.
8. Short, R. V. 1960. In *The Biosynthesis and Secretion of Adrenocortical Steroids* (F. Clark and J. K. Grant, eds.), Cambridge University Press, London.
9. Stylianou, M., Forchielli, E., and Dorfman, R. I. 1961. *J. Biol. Chem.* 236: 1318.
10. Stylianou, M., Forchielli, E., Tummillo, M., and Dorfman, R. I. 1961. *J. Biol. Chem.* 236: 692.

IV

Ralph I. Dorfman, Ph.D.
HIRSUTISM AND POLYCYSTIC OVARIES

This chapter is concerned with hirsutism as possibly related to polycystic ovaries. After definition of the syndrome the biosynthetic capabilities of normal ovaries will be discussed together with the biosynthetic modifications associated with these abnormal polycystic ovaries. A final section will deal with biochemical changes resulting from various therapeutic procedures.

DEFINITION

This chapter will deal especially with a variant of the Stein-Leventhal syndrome which includes patients who have two apparently related difficulties. These are hirsutism and/or virilism and polycystic ovaries. The patients may also have abnormalities of the menstrual cycle including ovulation.

THE NORMAL OVARY

The normal ovary possesses the potential of producing $C_{19}O_2$ androgens (Table 4-1), progesterone (Table 4-2), and estrogens (Table 4-3).

Some quantitative isolation studies on normal ovaries were reported by Mahesh and Greenblatt [56]. They isolated androst-4-ene-3,17-dione from normal human ovaries at the mean level of 0.9 μg per gram of tissue (Table 4-4). If the patient, just before surgery, was subjected to β-methasone suppression and stimulated with human pituitary follicle-stimulating hormones, 5.2 μg. of 17α-OH progesterone per g of ovary were detected together with 10 μg of androst-4-ene-3, 17-dione.

Table 4-1. Biosynthesis of Androgens by Ovaries

Substrate	Product	Test System	Species	References
Progesterone	Androst-4-ene-3,17-dione	Tumor homogenate	Human	Wiest, et al. [85]
Pregnenolone 17α-Hydroxy-progesterone	Androst-4-ene-3,17-dione (presumptive)	Normal & Stein-Leventhal	Human	Lanthier & Sandor [52]
17α-Hydroxy-progesterone	Androst-4-ene-3,17-dione	Slice	Human	Lanthier & Sandor [52A]
Progesterone	Androst-4-ene-3,17-dione	Minced	Human	Warren & Salhanick [84]
Progesterone 17α-Hydroxy-progesterone	Testosterone Androst-4-ene-3,17-dione	Homogenate	Human	Kase, et al. [46]
Progesterone	Androst-1,4-diene-3,17-dione	Ovary (polycystic)	Bovine	Gawienowski, et al. [21]
Acetate	Testosterone	Slices (Stein-Leventhal)	Human	Leon, et al. [54]
	Androst-4-ene-3,17-dione Dehydroepi-androsterone	Ovary (follicular cyst linings minced)	Human	Ryan & Smith [67]
	Testosterone Androst-4-ene 3,17-dione (preliminary)	Stein-Leventhal	Human	O'Donnell & McCaig [59]
Progesterone	Androst-4-ene-3,17-dione	Homogenate	Bovine	Solomon, et al. [78]
	Androst-4-ene-3,17-dione Testosterone	Arrhenoblastoma homogenate	Human	Savard, et al. [69]

CAUSATIVE AGENT OF HIRSUTISM

Testosterone is about 20 times more active than any of the other naturally occurring androgens, such as androst-4-ene-3,17-dione, 11β-hydroxyandrost-4-ene-,3, 17-dione and dehydroepian-drosterone. On this basis and for a variety of reasons which will be developed later, the hypothesis has been suggested that in the syndrome of hirsutism and polycystic ovaries, the concentration of testosterone

in the blood determines the intensity of the syndrome. The possibility
exists that other androgens, less active than testosterone, but in much
higher concentrations may be responsible for the clinical effect. If,
in fact, this should occur, it is expected that a proportionately high
level of 17-ketosteroids would be excreted and most likely there would
be a parallel increased plasma 17-ketosteroid concentration.

Table 4-2. Biosynthesis of Progesterone by Ovaries

Substrate	Test System	Species	References
Cholesterol	Corpora lutea in vitro	Bovine	Solomon, et al. [78]
Acetate	Ovarian Mince	Human Bovine	Sweat, et al. [81]
	Ovary (follicular cyst linings minced)	Human	Ryan & Smith [67]
20α–Hydroxy–cholesterol	Corpus luteum homogenate	Bovine	Tamaoki & Pincus [82]

The following published case illustrates that testosterone was
produced by a polycystic ovary which was associated with considerable
hirsutism while the 17-ketosteroid levels were essentially normal.
The study of this patient was an example in international cooperation.
Dr. Leon of Brazil treated the patient and did the incubation, and the
biochemical aspects were accomplished at the Worcester Foundation
in Shrewsbury, Massachusetts by Dr. Castro, a visiting scientist
from Lisbon, Portugal.

A 23-year old white woman was first admitted to the hospital on
May 21, 1956, at the age of 21. She had been moderately obese as a
child and continued to gain excessive weight after puberty. She had
noted the first signs of her disease at the age of 18.

Menarche was established at 12 followed by normal menstrual periods of three days' duration, although she had the impression that
the quantity of the menstrual flow had been scanty. Her general condition was satisfactory and her past history was not significant. She
had had mumps as a child. There was no hirsutism in the family. She
had acne.

At physical examination, the presence of excessive hair was noted
on the chin, in the mandibulary area, this being less along her superior
lip. Long, firm hair was present on her breasts and the abdominal
hair followed a masculine pattern. She had normal axillary hair and

her pubic hair spread to the anal region. Some slight white striae were present at both sides of the abdomen. Her musculature and bone configuration were normal. The thyroid gland was palpable but of normal consistency. Examination of the head, heart, lungs, lymphatic system, extremities, and neurologic system yielded nothing unusual.

Table 4-3. Biosynthesis of Estrogens by Ovaries

Substrate	Product	Test System	Species	References
Acetate	Estrone Estradiol-17β	Homogenate	Dog	Rabinowitz & Dowben [63]
			Human	Ryan & Smith [66]
			Various	Rabinowitz & Oleksyshyn [64]
Testosterone	Estradiol-17β	Slices	Human	Baggett, et al. [57] Hollander & Hollander [33]
	Estrone Estradiol-17β Estriol	Slices	Human	Wotiz, et al. [87]
	Estradiol-17β	Slice	Dog	Hollander & Hollander [32]
Androst-4-ene-3,17-dione	Estrone	Follicular fluid	Human Bovine	Meyer [57]
	Estrone Estradiol-17β	Follicular cyst linings homogenized	Human	Smith & Ryan [77]
Progesterone	Estrone Estradiol-17β	Mince	Human	Ryan & Smith [66]
		Idiopathic hirsutism	Human	Goldzieher & Axelrod [24]
Cholesterol	Estrone	Mince of follicular cyst linings	Human	Ryan & Smith [67]

The external genitalia were normal; no atrophy was seen on the labia majora or the labia minora. Her clitoris was small. Palpation was negative. At rectal examination a small uterus was found.

Height: 158 cm; weight: 63 kg; blood pressure: 130 x 80 mm Hg. Laboratory Findings: Slight estrogenic activity was noted by vaginal smears (30 per cent acidophilic cells at the thirteenth day of the menstrual cycle). She had tricomoniasis.

Blood electrolytes: Na 140 mEq/L:K 4.1 mEq/L:P 4.16 mg/100 ml; Ca 9.75 mg/100 ml; Cl 96 mEq/L.

Glucose tolerance test: 87, 141, 114, 101, 109 mg/100 ml.

Insulin tolerance test: 94, 49, 98, 101, 91 mg/100 ml.

There was a diminished iodine uptake (20.6 per cent) and a urine excretion of iodine of 61.9 per cent.

Basal metabolic rate: +2 -1.

Blood cholesterol: 149 mg/100 ml.

Urinary gonadotrophins: between 10 and 20 mu/24 hours.

17-Ketosteroids: 11.4 mg/24 hours.

11-Oxysteroids: 1.2-2.2 mg/24 hours.

Estrogenic substances: more than 16 r.u.

Table 4-4. Influence of Human FSH on the Concentration of Steroids in Normal Ovaries - Adrenals Suppressed with β-Methasone*

Type of ovary (treatment)	μg/gram of ovary			
	DHA	A	17α-OH P	17α-OH Preg
Normal	<0.8	1.1	<1.0	<1.0
Normal	<0.8	0.9	<1.0	<1.0
Normal	<0.8	0.8	<1.0	<1.0
Normal (β-methasone-HP-FSH)	<0.8	10.0	5.2	<1.0

*Mahesh & Greenblatt [56]

On November 13, 1957, the patient complained that her menstruations had become more scanty and that her hirsutism was more accentuated. A laparoscopy was done the next day and bilateral ovarian enlargement was noted, the ovaries being pale in color, suggesting Stein-Leventhal syndrome. The basal temperature was monophasic. The vaginal smears did not show more than 30 per cent acidophilic cells.

On July 16, 1958, a wedge resection was done on both ovaries. The right ovary was enlarged (4 x 3 cm) and had many microcysts on its surface. The left ovary was 3 x 2 cm and also had microcysts. Microscopic examination showed a thickened tunica albuginea and some fibrosis of the stroma, but follicles in all stages and some corpora albicantia were present. The 17-ketosteroids of the patient continued to be normal after the operation.

November 18, 1957: 8.27 mg/24 hours.

December 18, 1957: 8.12 mg/24 hours.

July 8, 1958: 10.98 mg/24 hours.

September 5, 1958: 11.41 mg/24 hours.

When the patient was seen two months after the operation, the menstruation was more regular. The menstrual flow was more abundant and accompanied by abdominal pain. The temperature curves had become diphasic. She lost some weight after the operation. Vaginal smears done after the operation were as follows:

August 4, 1958: 70 per cent acidophilic cells (menstruation on July 17).

August 12, 1958: 20 per cent acidophilic cells

September 2, 1958: 40 per cent acidophilic cells (fifteenth day since the menstruation).

Tissue slices from the resected portion of the polycystic ovary were incubated with 0.5 mC of sodium acetate-1-C^{14}, 10 ml of the patient's serum, 5 mg of glucose, 0.01 mMole of sodium fumarate with phosphate buffer at 37°C for 3.5 hours under oxygen. The mixture was homogenized and extracted successively with ethyl acetate, ether-chloroform (4:1), and acetone. The combined extracts were concentrated to dryness under a stream of nitrogen, and 10 mg each of testosterone and androst-4-ene-3, 17-dione were added to the dried residues. The residue, containing the added steroids, was partitioned between 90 per cent methanol and ligroin, and the methanolic fraction contained 95,000 counts per minute.

The neutral fraction, prepared by partition between toluene and 1 N sodium hydroxy, contained 37,500 counts per minute.

The testosterone and androst-4-3, 17-dione fractions were obtained by paper chromatography in the ligroin-propylene-glycol system. Radiochemical purity was not achieved with the eluted crystalline material having the mobility of androst-4-ene-3, 17-dione. The testosterone fraction was chromatographed on a silica gel column and in a Bush system (petroleum ether, benzene-methanol-water), and 0.5 mg of testosterone was obtained with a specific activity of 80 c/min/mg, which was considered to be radiochemically pure. This material was acetylated and chromatographed on paper, and the testosterone acetate was recrystallized to a constant specific activity of 79 c/min/mg (calculated as testosterone).

It is clear that testosterone can be formed by normal human ovaries, as has been demonstrated by Kase, et al. [46]. The qualitative detection of newly formed testosterone in this study, therefore, does not set off this Stein-Leventhal ovary from a normal ovary. The finding herein reported is consistent with the idea that hirsutism and even virilism related to abnormal ovaries may be due to a relatively small increased production of testosterone insufficient to produce a significant rise in urinary 17-ketosteroids.

In another study we were able to show that Stein-Leventhal ovaries (polycystic) were more efficient producers of testosterone than normal ovaries. The details of this study are described in the following section.

The tissue was finally minced, suspended in the appropriate co-factor solution based on tissue weight, and then homogenized in a Potter-Elvejhem type homogenizer. The homogenate was transferred, with the aid of an equal volume of isotonic potassium chloride, to incubation flasks containing progesterone-7-H^3, (specific activity 31 $\mu C/g$) and 17α-hydroxyprogesterone-4-C^{14} (specific activity of 44.7 $\mu C/mg$). The procedure was carried out at 4°C. Incubations were performed in open flasks with constant mixing for three hours at 37°C.

Each incubate was covered with a five-fold volume of ethyl acetate and allowed to stand overnight at 4°C. Debris was filtered and re-extracted three times with additional solvent. The combined extract was taken to dryness under reduced pressure. The dried extract was taken up in 70 per cent aqueous methanol and partitioned against petroleum ether twice for fat removal. Following back extraction of petroleum ether with fresh 70 per cent methanol, the aqueous methanol solutions were combined and concentrated to an aqueous sludge in vacuo and extracted three times with equal volumes of redistilled methylene chloride. The methylene chloride extracts were partitioned twice with one-third volume 1.0 N NaOH to remove phenolic compounds. The resulting methylene chloride extracts were washed with small volumes of water until the washings were neutral, then dried over anhydrous sodium sulfate and concentrated to dryness in vacuo; then dried residue was taken up in 10 ml of benzene.

The steroids were separated by the paper chromatographic systems ligroin-propylene-glycol and the cyclohexane:benzene-propylene glycol. Adsorption chromatography was also carried out using Woelm alumina (grade II) eluted with various ratios of benzene and petroleum ether.

The steroids were localized in dried paper strips by ultraviolet light scanning using authentic standards run on parallel strips. The zones were then eluted with methanol.

To facilitate radiochemical purity studies, testosterone was acetylated in the conventional manner overnight at room temperature with acetic anhydride and pyridine in the ratio of 1.2:1. For recovery of the testosterone the acetate was hydrolyzed overnight or refluxed for two hours in the presence of two equivalents of sodium hydroxide. Androst-4-ene-3,17-dione dioxime was formed by refluxing the free steroid in methanol containing sodium acetate and hydroxylamine hydrochloride.

All samples were analyzed for both tritium and C^{14} content in a Packard Tricarb liquid scintillation counter.

To the neutral fraction was added 10 mg of carrier androst-4-ene-3,17-dione and the mixture was chromatographed on paper in the ligroin-propylene glycol system. Similarly, 10 mg of carrier testosterone was added to the neutral extract and the mixture was chromatographed either in the ligroin-propylene glycol system for forty hours or for twenty-four hours in the cyclohexane:benzene-propylene glycol system. The testosterone zone was eluted, acetylated, extracted, and chromatographed on 300 mg of alumina. Crystalline material was obtained in the fractions eluted with 10 per cent benzene - 90 per cent petroleum ether. When necessary, this material was chromatographed on paper several times to achieve constant specific activity for the acetate. As a further test of radiochemical purity, the acetate was hydrolyzed and the free compound recrystallized to constant specific activity.

Androst-4-ene-3, 17-dione after elution from the paper was also chromatographed on a 300 mg alumina column. Crystalline material was consistently eluted with 20 per cent benzene - 80 per cent petroleum ether. In all instances, this material exhibited considerable purity on recrystallization from ether-petroleum ether. Following three crystallizations yielding material of constant specific activity, the dioxime was prepared. This derivative was recrystallized three times and again constant specific activity was obtained.

Table 4-5 summarizes the percentage conversion observed when normal and Stein-Leventhal ovaries were incubated with the substrate 17α-hydroxyprogesterone-4-C^{14}. Both testosterone and androst-4-ene-3, 17-dione were formed in all instances. Each of the androgens was produced in greater amounts by the abnormal tissue than by the normal tissue. The mean testosterone was 0.24 per cent and the androst-4-ene-3, 17-dione was 1.6 per cent for the normal tissue. By contrast, the Stein-Leventhal tissue produced 1.5 per cent of testosterone, an increase of six-fold and 21.5 per cent for androst-4-ene-3, 17-dione or an increase of about thirteen-fold.

Table 4-5. Conversion of 17α-Hydroxy-progesterone-4-C^{14} to Testosterone(T) and Androst-4-ene-3, 17-dione(A)

Tissue	Per cent conversion	
	T	A
Normal human Ovaries	0.31	2.2
	0.30	not completed
	0.11	0.89
Stein-Leventhal	0.49	10.0
	1.70	28.2
	0.4	7.1
	0.93	6.4
	2.72	55.8

Table 4-6 deals with the same tissues already discussed in Table 4-5 except that the substrate in these studies was progesterone-7α-H^{3}. The control (normal) ovaries produced a mean of 0.14 per cent of testosterone and 1.5 per cent of the weaker androgen, androst-4-ene-3, 17-dione. Again it was observed that each Stein-Leventhal ovary produced a greater amount of both testosterone and androst-4-ene-3, 17-dione. The testosterone formation was 0.95 per cent for the Stein-Leventhal ovaries while androst-4-ene-3, 17-dione was increased to 11.0 per cent.

Table 4-6. Conversion of Progesterone-7α-H^3 to Testosterone (T)
and Androst-4-ene-3, 17-dione (A)

Tissue	Per cent conversion	
	T	A
Normal human ovary	0.16	1.7
	0.15	1.3
	0.10	not completed
Stein-Leventhal human ovary	0.70	3.7
	1.08	15.7
	0.45	3.9
	0.43	2.6
	2.1	29.3

Consideration of the radioisotopic content of the newly formed testosterone and androst-4-ene-3, 17-dione demonstrated a striking difference in the amounts produced between the normal and abnormal tissue. The data also revealed the possibility of a new biosynthetic pathway directly from progesterone to testosterone. If the postulated pathway requiring androst-4-ene-3, 17-dione as the obligatory intermediate in testosterone biosynthesis was the only one operative, it would be expected that, assuming complete mixing of the two precursor substrates (one tritiated, the other C^{14}-labeled) the ratio of H^3/C^{14} would be the same in both the formed androst-4-ene-3, 17-dione and testosterone. Examination of the data indicates that the ratio of H^3/C^{14} was greater by three times in the Stein-Leventhal ovaries than in the normal tissue (Table 4-7). To explain this discrepancy, a second biosynthetic pathway is suggested whereby testosterone is formed directly from progesterone without 17α-hydroxyprogesterone and Δ^4-androstene-3, 17-dione as intermediates. Suggestive evidence for the existence of such an alternate pathway has been known for some years from microbiologic studies. Quite recently this transformation has been established by Fonken, et al. [18], who isolated testosterone acetate after the incubation of progesterone with *Cladosporium resinae*. These investigators further showed that the organism did not contain the enzyme necessary for acetylation of testosterone but that incubation of progesterone-21-C^{14} produced testosterone acetate with C^{14} in the methyl carbon of the acetate.

The suggested new biosynthetic pathway to testosterone may oper-
ate in varying degrees in all steroids-producing organs. Why one pathway should gain prominence over another, as appears to be the case in
these studies, has no satisfactory answer at this time. However, the
finding of a competitive interplay of biosynthetic pathways is consistent with the observations of Lindner on calf and bull testis. He found
that as the testis matured, a reversal of C_{19} androgen production occurred with a greater quantity of testosterone being produced.

Table 4-7.   Ratio of H^3/C^{14} in Testosterone (T) and Androst-4-ene-3,17-dione (A)
Biosynthesized from Progesterone-7α-H^3 and 17α-Hydroxyprogesterone-4-C^{14}

Tissue	H^3/C^{14}		
	T	A	$\dfrac{T}{A}$
Normal human ovary	0.52	0.78	0.67
	1.3	1.45	0.9
Stein-Leventhal ovary	1.4	0.37	3.8
	0.61	0.56	1.1
	1.1	0.55	2.0
	0.46	0.41	1.1
	0.77	0.53	1.5

Mean normal = 0.8
Mean S-L = 1.9

A variety of studies on human normal and Stein-Leventhal subjects
have been published in the last few years and will be discussed in this
section. In 1960 Lanthier and Sandor [52] wrote, "It is postulated that
Stein-Leventhal Syndrome may be caused, at least partially, by exag-
gerated formation of androst-4-ene-3, 17-dione or possibly by decreased aromatization of this androgenic steroid." Lanthier [5] studied the
urine of polycystic ovarian patients with hyperthecosis. In this paper
12 normal women had 17-ketosteroids of 7.5 ± 2.1 and the 27 Stein-
Leventhal patients had a mean value of 11.2 ± 3.7. The androsterone
and etiocholanolone fractions were significantly elevated. The author
concluded that he was unable to elucidate the role of the ovary versus
the adrenal in this syndrome.

Warren and Salhanick [84] reported an extensive study on steroid
biosynthesis by normal and Stein-Leventhal ovaries. The abnormal
ovaries incubated with progesterone yielded high amounts of 17α-
hydroxyprogesterone and androst-4-ene-3, 17-dione. The conclusion
was important but the possible role of testosterone was not mentioned:
"It is concluded that the cystic structures of the Stein-Leventhal ovary
have the capacity to synthesize greater amounts of recognized androgenic compounds than do normal ovaries."

Other groups who failed to find testosterone include Zander [89]
in human ovarian tissue, Short [75] in mare follicular fluid and Sweat,

et al. [81] who failed to detect testosterone in extracts from human and bovine corpus luteum.

In what appears to be a highly significant paper, Sandor and Lanthier [68] reported the incubation of androst-4-ene-3,17-dione with ovarian slices from normal patients and with Stein-Leventhal ovarian wedges for six and twenty-four hours in the presence of human chorionic gonadotropin. Both penicillin and streptomycin sulfate were added to the twenty-four-hour incubations to prevent bacterial contamination. The striking result of these incubations (Table 4-8) is the fact that the abnormal tissue had the facility to reduce the 17-ketone group so effectively, forming the highly active androgen, testosterone. Recently Sharma, et al. [73] observed a parallel phenomenon in that androst-4-ene-3,17-dione was more efficiently transformed to testosterone by adult rat testis homogenate than immature rat testis tissue preparations.

Table 4-8.   Formation of Testosterone from Androst-4-ene-3,17-dione by Incubation with Normal and Stein-Leventhal Ovaries*

Type of ovarian tissue	Incubation Time hours	Testosterone formation μg/g/hr.
Normal	6	0.28
Stein-Leventhal		1.52
Normal	24	1.15
Stein-Leventhal		2.28

*Sandor & Lanthier [68]

In an earlier section of this chapter it was indicated that the possible new biosynthetic pathway, progesterone to testosterone acetate to testosterone, provided a means to explain Linder's [54a] finding. The results of Sandor and Lanthier [68] and those of Sharma, et al. 73 also provide explanations for these data.

Axelrod and Goldzieher [4] (Table 4-9) found an increase in the biosynthetic yield of testosterone from 0.4 per cent for a single normal ovary to 1.1 per cent for the mean of seven polycystic glands. Five of the seven observations on the polycystic ovaries with respect to testosterone formation percentages were within what probably is the range for biosynthesis for the normal gland. On the other hand, the formation of androst-4-ene-3,17-dione was enormously increased from 1.1 per cent for the single control ovary to a mean of 25.1 per cent for the seven polycystic ovaries. Only one polycystic ovary was in what might be considered the normal range.

Table 4-9. Conversion of Progesterone of Testosterone (T)
and Androst-4-ene-3,17-dione (A)*

| Type of ovary | Per cent conversion | |
	T	A
Normal	0.4	1.1
Polycystic	2.2	22.6
	3.4	25.1
	0.5	8.9
	0.0	52.2
	0.7	7.6
	0.4	0.8
	0.5	58.6
Mean	1.1	25.1

* Axelrod & Goldzieher [4]

Mahesh and Greenblatt [56] (Table 4-10) have analyzed normal and polycystic ovaries for their steroid content as well as a polycystic ovary obtained from a patient who had been subjected to β-methasone and human pituitary follicle-stimulating hormone treatment. The comparative values indicate that the two polycystic ovaries were quite different in their steroid composition. One had a concentration of 6.4 μg of dehydroepiandrosterone per g but no increment in androst-4-ene-3,17-dione, nor could 17α-hydroxyprogesterone and 17α-hydroxypreg-nenolone be detected. In the other polycystic gland dehydroepiandros-terone was not elevated, but androst-4-ene-3,17-dione was increased more than twelve times and 17α-hydroxyprogesterone was detected but not 17α-hydroxypregnenolone.

Table 4-10. Comparative Steroid Concentrations of Normal
and Polycystic Ovaries

Type of ovaries (No. of subjects)	DHA	A	17α-OHP	17α-OH Preg.
Normal (3)	<0.8	0.9	<1.0	<1.0
Polycystic (2)[†]	<0.8	12.1	2.2	<1.0
	6.4	<0.5	<1.0	<1.0
Polycystic (1)[‡]	<0.8	4.5	1.8	<1.0

*Mahesh & Greenblatt [56]
†Hirsutism - Elevated - 17-KS
‡Hirsutism - Treatment β-methasone for six months + HP - FSH

A most interesting test for polycystic ovaries highly efficient in androgen production was by Nicolosi [58] who claims that the administration of progesterone does not influence the 17-ketosteroids of normal individuals but causes an increase in some women with idiopathic hirsutism and menstrual troubles, and in all patients with the Stein-Leventhal syndrome. It would appear that the ovaries of these women can remove enough progesterone from circulation to express the higher androgen-producing capabilities of these glands.

CONCENTRATION OF TESTOSTERONE IN PLASMA

The concentration of testosterone in the plasma of hirsute women with polycystic ovarian disease has been discussed in Chapter 2. These studies establish the possibility of testosterone being the causative agent. This point is made clearer if we examine the relative potencies of naturally occurring androgens in man.

RELATIVE POTENCIES OF NATURALLY OCCURRING ANDROGENS IN MAN AND TESTOSTERONE PRODUCTION RATES

What are the substances that really bring about the full sexual development in men and what are the substances that produce hirsutism and virilism in the female? An aid to the solution of the problem would be a knowledge of the relative androgenicity of these agents in man, and here our knowledge is limited. It is known that testosterone administered by injection in an amount of 100 mg per month will cause slight hirsutism in some women, but not all. If, however, the dose is increased to about 200 mg per month, or about 6 mg a day, definite masculinization occurs. When 200 to 400 milligrams of testosterone were administered per month to women with metastatic breast cancer, hirsutism and hoarseness were observed within one month in 20 per cent of the patients. In seven months this dosage produced an incidence of 90 per cent of hirsutism. On this basis, one may say that an endogenous production of 6 mg of testosterone per day over a period of months will probably reproduce the signs of hirsutism in women and at the level of 12 mg per day of production of testosterone, true virilism would be observed.

In addition to testosterone, androst-4-ene-3,17-dione, 11β-hydroxyandrost-4-ene-3,17-dione and dehydroepiandrosterone are known to be produced and to be present in the blood. Androst-4-ene-3,17-dione, at a dose of 300 mg every six or seven days caused mild facial hair growth in two patients and a slight voice change in a third woman of a group of ten women in a two- to three-month period. Since 7-14 mg per day of testosterone causes about the same effect [13], it is concluded that androst-4-ene-3, 17-dione in humans is about 5 per cent as active as testosterone.

Segaloff, et al. [71] have administered 100 mg of dehydroepian-drosterone three times per week without observing any virilism during periods of treatment up to 100 days.

Studies on the urinary excretion of 17-ketosteroids in men and women have indicated that although there is considerable overlap in individual values of 17-ketosteroids between men and women, there is nonetheless a consistent significant difference in the mean excretion values. This is illustrated in Table 4-11, which represents values taken from five representative studies. Two striking points are illustrated: (1) that the values within any single group vary by as much as four-fold from the highest value to the lowest one in a group, and (2) that the difference between mean values of men and women only varies from 3.2 to 4.4 mg per day. If one assumes the value of 4.0 mg as the mean net difference between men and women, then a rough estimate of testosterone production would be of the order of 8 mg. Since testosterone administration results in a 50 per cent recovery in the urine as androsterone and etiocholanolone, this would mean that the 4 mg of extra 17-ketosteroids in the male may represent approximately 8 mg of endogenous 17-ketosteroid precursor, that is, testosterone. Thus

Table 4-11. Representative Urinary 17-Ketosteroid (17 KS) Excretion Values for Men and Women

Fraction analyzed	Men			Women			Difference in 17-KS between men and women
	No. of subjects	Age range (year)	Mean urinary 17-KS mg/day (range)	No. of subjects	Age range (year)	Mean urinary 17-KS mg/day (range)	
Total Neutral Corrected	28	20–30	14.4 (5.5-25.2)	20	20–30	10.0 (4-16)	4.4
Total Neutral Corrected	13	20–40	14.2 (9.8-20.8)	15	20–40	10.2 (5.8-17.0)	4.0
Total Neutral Corrected	73	24–42	12.5 (6.7-27.2)	65	23–37	8.2 (3.8-16.9)	4.3
Total Neutral Corrected	14	20–40	13.6 (6.0-2.8)	18	20–35	10.0 (4.8-17.0)	3.6
Ketonic	40	20–40	10.2 (4.9-18.4)	18	20–40	7.0 (1.5-9.7)	3.2

the hypothesis could be suggested that the 8 mg of testosterone produces the necessary development in a man and that this amount of testosterone in a woman would produce significant virilization.   Thus far
we have assumed that all of the extra 17-ketosteroids in men are derived from testosterone.   But since the testis also produces a reasonable amount of androst-4-ene-3,17-dione, it is quite likely that the
figure of 8 mg of testosterone per day is high and must be reduced by
a factor to account for the testis production of androst-4-ene-3,17-
dione.   On this basis, the value of 8 mg of testosterone per day in the
male would be a reasonable upper limit for daily production [12].

The recommended dose of testosterone for adequate replacement
therapy in male hypogonadism varies with the type of preparation the
daily production estimate on this basis employed, but, in general, is
of the same order as would be expected from previous calculations.
As the propionate injected in oil, 75 mg of testosterone per week or
10 mg per day ensures adequate therapy.   For a long-acting ester such
as testosterone β-cyclopentylpropionate, a single dose of 200-300 mg
is adequate for three weeks, which would be of the order of 10 to 15
mg per day.   When testosterone is employed as a pellet implant, about
10 mg per day is required.

17-KETOSTEROIDS IN OVARIAN TISSUE

Trace, et al. [83] (Table 4-12) studies 17-ketosteroids in ovarian
tissue from normal and polycystic ovarian patients with and without

Table 4-12. Concentration of 17-Ketosteroids in Normal Ovaries and
from Patients with Polycystic Ovaries with and without Hirsutism*

Type of ovary	Hirsutism	No. of subjects	Mean 17-ketosteroids in ovarian tissue μg/g (range)
Normal	No	5	4.0 (1.9-7.8)
Normal	Yes	1	2.0
Stein-Leventhal	Yes	10	3.7 (1.2-8.6)
Stein-Leventhal	Yes (also clitorial enlargement)	3	1.9 (1.6-2.3)
Stein-Leventhal	No	3	8.1 (7.4-8.6)

*Trace, et al. [83]

hirsutism. No correlation between the 17-ketosteroids in the tissue and the clinical state could be established.

OVARIAN AND PERIPHERAL VEIN BLOOD

Seeman and Saracino [70] studied the concentrations of 17-keto-steroids in ovarian vein and peripheral blood as well as peripheral blood after bilateral castration and wedge resection. Peripheral blood was found to contain between 17 and 120 μg of 17-ketosteroid per 100 ml of plasma, while ovarian vein plasma 17-ketosteroids varied from 40 to 475 μg. The mean difference was 138 ± 38.1 μg per 100 ml plasma.

Ovariectomy caused an impressive change in the titer of peripheral 17-ketosteroids (Table 4-13).

Table 4-13. Influence of Ovariectomy on Peripheral
Plasma Total 17-Ketosteroids*

	17-KS μg/100 ml	
Before	After (no. of days)	Difference
55	28 (12)	-27
	5 (24)	-50
	25 (44)	-30
53	3 (14)	-54
41	17 (15)	-24
85	57 (7)	-28

*Seeman & Saracino [70]

Preliminary studies on testosterone production rates are now available and indicate that the highly active androgen is produced at the rate of from 4.1 to 8.8 mg per day in men [34]. Between twelve and forty-four days after surgery the peripheral plasma 17-ketoster-oids decreased from 50 to 90 per cent of the presurgical level.

The peripheral plasma 17-ketosteroid values of patients subjected to wedge resection showed significant decreases as indicated in the representative figures in Table 4-14.

STEROIDS IN HIRSUTE-POLYCYSTIC OVARIAN PATIENTS

Pregnanetriolone

Pregnanetriolone, a steroid which is excreted in excessive amounts in patients with congenital adrenal hyperplasia [17] and in patients with the milder form of this disease manifested after puberty [7] is absent from normal urine (less than 1 μg per day) [16]. This steroid has now been found in 16 consecutive patients having the Stein-Leventhal syndrome [74]. These patients, showing infertility, menstrual irregularities and hirsutism, excreted pregnanetriolone at the rate of 8 to 200 μg per day while other steroid indices were normal; 17-ketosteroids - 11.4 mg ± 2.72 mg, 17-ketogenic steroids - 6.8 mg ± 2.1 mg, pregnanediol ± 1.2 mg ± 0.3 mg (normal for follicular phase); urinary estrogens in four subjects was within the normal range usually found before the ovulation peak, and pregnanetriol levels were normal, on the basis of results previously published by Cox [10] and Goldzieher and Axelrod [25].

Cox and Shearman [11] studied six hirsute Stein-Leventhal women. These authors find less than 10 μg per day of pregnanetriolone in the urine of their normal women, but all six of the hirsute patients had 40 to 140 μg of this steroid per day before and after wedge resection.

Table 4-14. Biosynthesis of Estrogens by Normal and Polycystic Ovaries*

Subject (no.)	Per cent formation from progesterone added (range)		
	Biosynthesis of 19-oxygenated C_{19} steroids	Biosynthesis of estrogens	
		Estrone	Estradiol-17β
Normal (1)	3.9	0	4.8
Polycystic ovaries (7)	30.1† (1.2-67.8)	0	0.98 (0-5.9)

*Data from five subjects, results from remaining two not available.
†Axelrod & Goldzieher [4]

This study [11] also reports an increased pregna-5-ene-3β,17α, 20α-triol excretion in the hirsute patients. Normal women excreted a mean of 0.12 (0.06-0.21) mg per day of this Δ^5-3β-hydroxy steroid, while the mean value for the Stein-Leventhal patients (before or after wedge resection) was 0.41 (0.24-0.89) mg per day.

Estrogen Metabolism

Axelrod and Goldzieher [3], [4] find that human polycystic ovarian tissues have a relatively deficient ability to produce aromatization, to produce 17α-hydroxylation, and to convert Δ^5-3β-hydroxy steroids to the Δ^4-3-ketosteroid. This is claimed to cause a failure in estrogen biosynthesis (Table 4-14) and an accumulation of testosterone, dehydroepiandrosterone and other C_{19} "metabolites." This theory had been previously suggested by Sandor and Lanthier [52], [52a] but seems to be inadequate as an explanation for the increase in "effective androgens."

Since the daily production of all $C_{19}O_2$ (androgens) per day is of the order of 20 mg per day, and since the daily estrogen production is probably of the order of 150 μg, it would be difficult to understand how this relatively minute amount of extra $C_{19}O_2$ (that portion that would not be aromatized) could be a factor of such importance.

The paper of Axelrod and Goldzieher [4] fails to mention the studies of Short [76], who studied the estrogen content of cystic fluid derived from both normal and Stein-Leventhal ovaries. This investigator found an increased amount of androst-4-ene-3,17-dione in Stein-Leventhal fluid (Table 4-15) compared to the concentration of that obtained in this steroid in the cystic fluid from normal ovaries. On the other hand, estradiol-17β was detected at the level of 4-156 μg per 100 ml of fluid from normal ovaries but none in Stein-Leventhal ovaries. These findings would indicate that these ovaries might be deficient estrogen formers. Other studies in this area do not support this conclusion.

Table 4-15. Androgen and Estrogen Production in Normal (N)
and Stein-Leventhal (S-L) Ovaries*

Compound	Source of cystic fluid	Conc. μg/100 ml
-4-Androst-ene-3,17-dione	N(7) S-L(5)	4-78 88-196
Estradiol-17β	N(7) S-L	4-156 not detected

*Short [76]

The concentration of the three estrogens, estrone, estradiol-17β and estriol, were analyzed by paper chromatography [49]. The Stein-Leventhal ovarian wedges contained significantly more estradiol-17β and estrone than was found in normal ovaries removed from the ninth to twenty-sixth day of the cycle (Table 4-16). These data are in harmony with the blood estrogen determinations reported from our laboratory and discussed in Chapter 1.

Jayle, et al. [41] clearly showed that estrogen excretion by "hairy virilized" women was not low compared to that of normal women during the luteal phase of the menstrual cycle and was significantly greater than that of ammenorrheic non-hirsute women. Shearman, et al. [74] reported normal estrogen levels in the urine of hirsute Stein-Leventhal patients.

Androsterone and Etiocholanolone

Androsterone and etiocholanolone are metabolites of both the highly active androgen testosterone and the weaker androgens androst-4-ene-3,17-dione and dehydroepiandrosterone and to a most limited extent of the non-androgens 17α-hydroxyprogesterone and 11-deoxycortisol. In view of these complications, it is not necessarily required that androsterone and etiocholanolone be increased in the hirsute patient. Studies dealing with this possibility have been published. Goldzieher and Green [26] summarized the results of sixty-two cases where the urinary 17-ketosteroids were separated so that a judgment may be made on the androsterone and etiocholanolone titers. In the urines of slightly more than half of these patients these two steroids were elevated. Brooksbank [8] has received about seventeen papers, all of which indicated some increases in androsterone, etiocholanolone, or both, in hirsute women. The increase, when it occurred, did not pinpoint the androgen or androgens that were increased.

Table 4-16. Estrogens in Human Ovaries*

Subjects (age range)	No.	Remarks	μg/g Tissue (range)		
			Estrone	Estradiol-17β	Estriol
Normal (34–45)	4	9th to 26th day of cycle	0.54 (0.2–1.0)	0.62 (0.5–0.7)	0.24 (0–0.6)
Stein–Leventhal (25–35)	5		0.73 (0.5–1.5)	1.63 (1.1–2.5)	0.14 (0–0.9)
Pregnancy (28–40)	7	16–60 days	2.13 (0.6–4.2)	2.70 (0.5–10.6)	5.00 (0–18.9)

*Kecskes, et al. [49]

Dehydroepiandrosterone

About 37 per cent of a total of over 350 patients excreted an excessive amount of dehydroepiandrosterone (Table 4-17). In one group of about 100 patients not included in Table 4-17, a similar urinary increase in this steroid was observed in a high proportion of the cases. Goldzieher and Green [26] and Brooksbank [8] have reviewed the change in dehydroepiandrosterone recently.

Etiology

Gemzell, et al. [22] studied hirsute women who were divided into the following groups:
  I.   Normal menses, normal 17-KS and hirsute (100 women - 51 per cent).
  II. Menstrual irregularities, normal 17-KS-hirsute (65 women - 33 per cent).

Table 4-17.   Hirsutism Excretion of Dehydroepiandrosterone (DHA)

No. of patients	Results	Investigator
7	DHA increased in all (17-KS normal in 4)	Gardner [20]
Ca 100	High proportion of DHA	Audit & Boussemart [2] Karl [48] Lipsett & Riter [55] Sendrail, et al. [72] Zacco, et al. [9]
33	Only one had an increased DHA excretion	Devis [11a]
78	17 of 78 DHA increased	Jailer & Vande Wiele [39]
180	80 normal 17-KS but 23 had high DHA _____ 100 increased 17-KS and 75 had high DHA	Jayle, et al. [40]
4	3/4 increased	Gallagher, et al. [19]
56	7/56 increased	Goldzieher & Green [26]

III.   Elevated 17-KS with and without menstrual disorders and
       hirsute.
    The onset of symptoms at the age of 20 or younger was 50 per
cent for Group I, 62 per cent for II and 65 per cent for III.   These
values are hardly significantly different among each other.   There
were signs of ovulation after wedge resection in all groups: 70 per
cent for I, 35 per cent for II and 56 per cent for III.   Three of seven
patients studied in Group III had increases in dehydroepiandrosterone.

ETIOLOGY OF THE POLYCYSTIC-HIRSUTISM SYNDROME

    Allen and Woolf [1] suggested that the syndrome may be explained
on a genetic basis in which the medullary tissue of the ovary produced
an excessive quantity of androgens.   Testosterone in relatively small
amounts could cause the abnormality and they suggest that removal of
the medulla of the ovary may correct the difficulties by lowering the
androgen production.
    Pituitary gonadotropins have been implicated in the syndrome.
Luteotrophic hormone has been eliminated as prime cause on the basis
of corpora lutea in by far the great majority of cases.   In a detailed

study [35], [36], the FSH of 26 patients was studied. Normal values were found in 22, one was low and three slightly increased.

Luteinizing hormone (LH) may be implicated in the syndrome, but the relationship has not been vigorously established. Keetel, et al. [50] found increased titers of LH in the urine of bilateral polycystic ovaries. Greenblatt [27] has reported the same findings, as have Ingersoll and McDermott 35a . The latter report includes some suggestion that after surgery there was a return to normal LH excretion in two of five patients.

Although considerable difficulties attend the precise evaluation of urinary gonadotropin studies, the tendency is to believe that the majority of hirsute-polycystic patients have normal values [36].

THEORIES OF THE POLYCYSTIC OVARY-HIRSUTISM SYNDROME

Greenblatt [28] suggests that abnormal steroid biosynthesis may take place either in the ovary or in the adrenal, and that cases of adrenal origin may respond to corticoid therapy but not to ovarian resection. Cases of ovarian origin may respond either to reduction in ovarian mass by surgical means, to corticoid administration, or to both. Greenblatt [28] further comments that ovulation does not take place because of less LH per unit of ovarian mass, and his analysis does not include a definitive statement on androgens.

Hendrick [31] has speculated on the mechanism of corticoid therapy in women with anovulation, infertility, some hirsutism, and elevated 17-ketosteroids. One patient's urinary 17-ketosteroids were 35.4 mg per day; when treated with prednisolone, they became 5 mg per day; for 60 days the level fell to 3.3 mg and menses became normal followed by a normal pregnancy. A second patient, also hirsute, had a 17-ketosteroid value of 36.5 mg and on the same treatment the 17-ketosteroids fell in 90 days to 23.7, menses became normal, and a normal pregnancy ensued.

The authors say that the defect is in the adrenal gland and that inadequate levels of "cortisone" are produced. This causes an increased secretion of ACTH, increased androgens, depression of FSH, and resultant drop in ovarian function. Prednisolone corrects by suppression of ACTH. The cases chosen by Hendrick are not particularly good for his theory since one patient showed a good suppression, which was not true of the second patient, yet both gave good clinical effects. A second objection to this theory is the fact that it is conceivable to get a considerable reduction in the weak androgens without influencing the strong androgen testosterone and therefore producing no change in the causative agent of the hirsutism.

The studies of Jailer and Vande Weile [39] are of interest with respect to hirsutism. They judged seventeen patients to have hirsutism associated with an adrenal abnormality because the urinary 17-keto-steroids were elevated, because the urinary excretion of dehydro-epiandrosterone was increased, and because cortisone treatment was accompanied by a fall in urinary 17-ketosteroids and dehydroepian-drosterone disappeared. In another 27 patients there was evidence of polycystic ovaries and the urinary 17-ketosteroids were normal. Treatment with cortisone to four patients of this group was without effect on the menstrual cycle and on the 17-ketosteroid excretion pat-tern, but no data were given. The fact that dehydroepiandrosterone may be produced by the ovary tends to indicate that these explanations are most likely too simple.

Evans and Riley [14] advanced the idea that the anterior pituitary secretes sufficient FSH to cause an accumulation of atretic follicles, which results in polycystic ovaries because there is insufficient LH for luteinization. The result is oligomenorrhea and amenorrhea.

THERAPY

Effective treatment of the syndrome, including menstrual irregu-larity and sterility with or without hirsutism, was discovered by Stein and Leventhal [79] and Stein, et al. [80]. They suggested treatment by wedge resection, which restored normal menstrual cycles in about 80 per cent of the patients, and some 65 per cent of the infertile patients became pregnant within a few months of the surgery. Wedge resection has been practiced extensively since the announcement of this remark-able discovery. The return of regular cycles in 219 patients so treated, summarized from the literature, is recorded by Goldzieher and Green [26], for an average incidence for the series of 85 per cent. This does not include the Stein, et al. [79] series, but did include the reports of many investigators [1, 6, 9, 14, 30, 37, 38, 53, 60, 61]. Goldzieher and Green [26] reported on 39 cases of their own and found a return of 58 per cent.

The pregnancy figures were also collected from published cases by Goldzieher and Green [26] and these indicated that in the total of 466 patients recorded, 67 per cent became pregnant, while in the Goldzieher and Green [26] series the incidence was 33 per cent. The Stein, et al. [80] group was not included in the Goldzieher and Green [26] tabulation, and the percentage for this group was 65 per cent.

On the basis of four studies [1, 14, 61, 62] only nine per cent of 161 patients showed improvement in their hirsutism. The results of these studies are not far different from the observations by Goldzieher and Green [26] on thirty-nine patients where no change in hirsutism was noted. The data of Plate [62a] indicate a reasonable improvement in hirsutism in his Group III (Table 4-18).

It is most likely that wedge resection causes a decrease in hor-mone production which, in turn, seems to be a mechanism by which

Table 4-18. The Influence of Wedge Resection*

Type of patient (group no.)	No.	Improvement Per cent (fraction)		
		Hirsutism	Regular ovulatory cycles	Pregnancy
Regular ovulatory bleeding (I)	9	25 (1/4)		
Alternately ovulation & anovulatory bleeding (II)	18	14 (1/7)	83 (15/18)	33 (3/9)
Anovulatory bleeding (III)	61	22 (5/23)	62 (36/58)	45 (14/31)
Secondary amenorrhea (IV)	27	0 (0/9)	30 (8/27)	15 (3/20)
Primary amenorrhea (V)	8	0 (0/2)	38 (3/8)	0 (0/2)
Total		16 (7/45)	56 (62/111)	32 (20/62)

*Plate [62a]

the pituitary-ovarian cycle is stimulated for the menses to be regularized. Our studies reported in Chapter 2 clearly show that wedge resection on three occasions decreased the plasma testosterone 0.42 µg, 0.43 µg, and 0.36 µg per 100 ml respectively. We have referred earlier to the data of Seeman and Saracino [70] on plasma 17-ketosteroids. A clear difference in plasma 17-ketosteroids was observed as a result of wedge resection (Table 4-19).

Table 4-19. Peripheral Influence of Ovarian Wedge Resection on Plasma 17-Ketosteroids*

Before resection	17-KS g/100 ml after resection (no. of days)	Difference
300	72 (7)	-228
123	19 (9)	-104
133	44 (6)	- 89
109	34 (5)	- 75

*Seeman & Saracino [70]

A second form of therapy is corticoid treatment (see Chapter 7). It may be immediately noted that adequate corticoid therapy causes a drop in testosterone in blood of the same magnitude as seen after wedge resection. In the admitted small series the decrease was 0.35 μg, 0.37 μg and 0.09 μg when the initial value was 0.11.

Corticoids are an effective treatment in certain patients whose chief complaint is infertility. In a study dealing with this form of therapy in infertility associated with hirsutes and oligomenorrhea, Ferriman, Purdic, and Tindall [15] reported that seven or eight patients became pregnant, of which six ended in successful deliveries. Similar findings have been reported by many other groups, many earlier than the latter study [23, 29, 42, 43, 44, 45, 86].

ADRENAL ANDROGENIC HYPERFUNCTION

A number of investigators have suggested that a syndrome exists involving the adrenal and is expressed by certain androgenic effects including infertility. Zenner [90] has summarized the syndrome (adrenal androgenic hyperfunction and infertility) as involving: (1) infertility; (2) dysfunction resulting in anovulation, menstrual irregularity, or amenorrhea and hypoplasia of the sex-linked organs; and (3) hirsutism, acne, and other metabolic changes. Zenner [90] further suggests that this may be a form of the adrenogenital syndrome and that the causative factors were related to excessive amounts of adrenal androgens. The 17-ketosteroids could be elevated or normal with a shift in the components of the 17-ketosteroid group, as shown by paper chromatography.

Treatment with corticoids or a progestational agent corrected the infertility of these patients, as was evidenced by a significant number of pregnancies. Zenner also reports decreases in the hirsutism. The action of the corticoids, cortisol, and triamcinolone is explained on the basis of suppression of ACTH, which lessens androgen production by the adrenal gland. 17α-hydroxyprogesterone caproate was as effective as the corticoids in the treatment of the infertility and hirsutism, and this is explained by Zenner [90] on the basis of excessive repression of the LH which stimulated the adrenal. Another possible explanation would accept the idea of an increased amount of LH but would maintain that the stimulation was on the ovary and that the progestational agent relieved this stimulation and subsequently lowered the androgen production. Further, in the untreated patients with normal or slightly elevated 17-ketosteroid titers the causative agent is a small but significantly increased titer of testosterone.

Zenner's striking results are summarized in Tables 4-20 and 4-21.

Rakoff [65] indicated that cyclic administration of estrogens and progesterone "has not often proved to be effective in the usual case of

Stein-Leventhal Syndrome." Progesterone is claimed to be of value in treatment of polycystic ovaries in cases of hyper-estronism without hirsutism or vililization. A possible therapeutic course was the intramuscular injection of 250 mg of 17a-hydroxyprogesterone caproate at four-week intervals for a three- to six-month period followed by a rest period for re-evaluation.

Table 4-20. Results of Treatment of Infertility in Cases of Adrenal Androgenic Hyperfunction†

Treatment	Total no. of patients	No. of patients not pregnant (%)	Pregnant patients			
			No. (%)	No. of pregnancies	Normal No. (%)	Nonviable No. (%)
Cortril	26	7 (26.9)	19 (73.1)	22	12 (54.5)	10 (45.5)
Delalutin	44*	7 (19.5)	29 (80.5)	37	27 (72.9)	10 (27.1)
Kenacort	31	5 (16.2)	26 (83.8)	28	22 (78.9)	6 (21.1)

*Eight patients did not complete course of treatment.

†Zenner [90]

Table 4-21. Results of Treatment of Virilism and Other Disturbances †

Symptom	Cortril (N=53)		Delalutin (N=83)		Kenacort (N=86)	
	I	U*	I	U	I	U
Acne	22		23	2	29	
Hirsutism	11		19		32	1
Anovulation	25		44	3+	43	
Irr. menses	8	1	34	4+	36	
Amenorrhea	6		3	3+	4	1
General metabolic	8		3		10	
TOTAL	80	1	142	12 (10+)	154	2

*I = Improved; U = Unimproved
+Responded to Kenacort

†Zenner [90]

Rakoff [65] has reported that patients may obtain prompt improvement with low-dosage irradiation of the ovary. This therapy is said to be of little benefit in patients with persistently high FSH levels or with definite elevation of 17-ketosteroids.

REFERENCES

1. Allen, W. M., and Woolf, R. B. 1959. *Am. J. Obstet. & Gynec.* **77**: 826.
2. Audit, J. F., and Baussemart, E. 1954. *Press Med.* **62**: 1112.
3. Axelrod, L. R., and Goldzieher, J. W. 1962. *Arch. Biochem. Biophys.* **95**: 547.
4. Axelrod, L. R., and Goldzieher, J. W. 1962. *J. Clin. Endocrinol. & Metab.* **22**: 431.
5. Baggett, B., Engel, L. L., and Savard, K. 1956. *J. Biol. Chem.* **221**: 931.
6. Bailey, K. V. 1959. *J. Obstet. Gynaec. Brit. Emp.* **66**: 556.
7. Brooks, R. V., Mattingly, D., Mills, A. H., and Prunty, F. T. G. 1960. *Brit. Med. J.* **1**: 1294.
8. Brooksbank, B. W. L. 1961. *Physiol. Rev.* **41**: 623.
9. Buxton, C. L. and VandeWiele, R. 1954. *New England J. Med.* **251**: 293.
10. Cox, R. I. 1960. *Acta Endocrinol.* **33**: 447.
11. Cox, R. I., and Shearman, R. P. 1961. *J. Clin. Endocrinol. & Metab.* **21**: 586.
11a Devis, R. 1951. *Ann. Endocrinol.* **12**: 451.
12. Dorfman, R. I. 1960. First Intern. Congr. Endocrinol., Copenhagen Abstr. Symposia, Lectures and Round Table, Discussions, 211.
13. Dorfman, R. I., and Shipley, R. A. 1956. I: *Androgens, Biochemistry, Physiology, and Clinical Significance.* John Wiley and Sons, New York.
14. Evans, T. N., and Riley, G. M. 1960. *Am. J. Obstet. & Gynecol.* **80**: 873.
15. Ferriman, D., Purdie, A. W., and Tindall, W. J. 1961. *Brit. Med. J.* i: 1806.
16. Finkelstein, M. 1959. *Acta Endocrinol.* **30**: 489.
17. Finkelstein, M. 1962. I: *Methods in Hormone Research* (R. I. Dorfman, ed.) Vol. II, 169, Academic Press, New York.
18. Fonken, G. S., Murray, H. C., and Reineke, L. M. 1960. *J. Am. Chem. Soc.* **82**: 5507.
19. Gallagher, T. F., Kappos, A., Hellman, L., Lipsett, M. B., Pearson, O. H., and West, C. D. 1958. *J. Clin. Inv.* **37**: 794.
20. Gardner, L. I. 1953. *J. Clin. Endocrinol. & Metab.* **13**: 1054.
21. Gawienowski, A. M., Lee, S. L., and Marion, G. B. 1961. *Endocrinology* **69**: 388.
22. Gemzell, G. A., Tielinger, K. G., and Westman, A. 1959. *Endocrinology* **30**: 387.
23. Gold, J. J., and Frank, R. 1958. *Am. J. Obstet. & Gynecol.* **75**: 1034.
24. Goldzieher, J. W., and Axelrod, L. R. 1960. First Internat. Congr. Endocrinol., Copenhagen, July, 1960, 617.

25. Goldzieher, J.W., and Axelrod, L.R. 1962. *J. Clin. Endocrinol. & Metab.* 22: 425.
26. Goldzieher, J.W., and Green, J.A. 1962. *J. Clin. Endocrinol. & Metab.* 22: 325.
27. Greenblatt, R.B. 1951. *Postgrad. Med.* 9: 492.
28. Greenblatt, R.B. 1961. *Maryland State Med. J.* March, 1.
29. Greenblatt, R.B., Barfeld, W.E., and Lampros, C.R. 1956. *Fertil. & Steril.* 7: 203.
30. Haas, R.I., and Riley, G.M. 1955. *Am. J. Obstet. & Gynecol.* 70: 657.
31. Hendrick, J.W. 1961. *J. Florida Med. Assoc.* 48: 346.
32. Hollander, N., and Hollander, V.P. 1958. *J. Biol. Chem.* 233: 1097.
33. Hollander, N., and Hollander, V.P. 1959. *Cancer Res.* 19: 290.
34. Hudson, B. 1962. *Endocrine Society Program,* 16.
35. Ingersoll, F.M. In *Progress in Gynaecology,* Grune and Stratton, New York.
35a Ingersoll, F.M., and McArthur, J.W. 1959. *Am. J. Obstet. & Gynecol.* 77: 795.
36. Ingersoll, F.M., and McDermott, W.M. Jr. 1950. *Am. J. Obstet. & Gynecol.* 60: 117.
37. Jackson, R.L., and Dockerty, M.B. 1957. *Am. J. Obstet. & Gynecol.* 73: 161.
38. Jailer, J.W., and Vande Wiele, R.L. 1954. *Bull. Soc. belge Gynecol.* 24: 231.
39. Jailer, J.W., and Vande Wiele, R.L. 1954. *Gynaecologia* 138: 276.
40. Jayle, M.F., Malassis, D., and Pinaud, H. 1959. *Acta Endocrinol.* 31: 1.
41. Jayle, M.F., Scholler, R., Mauvais-Jarvis, P., and Metay, S. 1961. *Acta Endocrinol.* 36: 375.
42. Jefferies, W. McK., and Levy, R.R. 1959. *J. Clin. Endocrinol. & Metab.* 19: 1069.
43. Jefferies, W. McK., Weir, W.C., Weir, D.R., and Prouty, R.L. 1955. *Fertil. & Steril.* 9: 145.
44. Jones, G.E.S., and Jones, H.W. 1954. *Fertil. & Steril.* 6: 140.
45. Jones, G.E.S., Howard, J.E., and Langford, H. 1953. *Fertil. & Steril.* 4: 49.
46. Kase, N., Forchielli, E., and Dorfman, R.I. 1961. *Acta Endocrinol.* 37: 19.
47. Kase, N., Forchielli, E., and Dorfman, R.I. 1963, unpublished.
48. Karl, H.J. 1960. *Klin. Wochshr.* 38: 634.
49. Kecskes, L., Mutschler, F., Than, E., and Farkas, I. 1962. *Acta Endocrinol.* 39: 483.
50. Keetel, W.C., Bradbury, J.T., and Stoddard, F.J. 1957. *Am. J. Obstet. & Gynecol.* 73: 954.

51. Lanthier, A. 1960. *J. Clin. Endocrinol. & Metab.* 20: 1587.
52. Lanthier, A., and Sandor, T. 1960. *Metabolism* 9: 861.
52a Lanthier, A., and Sandor, T. 1960. *Laval Med.* 30: 624.
53. Lanthier, A., Lauze, S., and Gregnon, C.E. 1960. *Am. J. Med. Sci.* 239: 585.
54. Leon, A., Castro, M., and Dorfman, R.I. 1962. *Acta Endocrinol.* 39: 411.
54a Lindner, H.R. 1959. *Nature* 183: 4675.
55. Lipsett, M.B., and Riter, B. 1960. *Klin. Wochshr.* 20: 180.
56. Mahesh, V.B., and Greenblatt, R.B. 1962. *Endocrinology* 22: 441.
57. Meyer, A.S. 1955. *Biochim. Biophys. Acta* 24: 1435.
58. Nicolosi, G. 1960. *Progress Med.* (Napoli) 16: 238.
59. O'Donnell, V.J., and McCraig, J.G. 1959. *Biochem. J.* 71: 9P.
60. Personen, S., Timonsen, S., and Raili, M. 1959. *Acta Endocrinol.* 30: 405.
61. Phillip, E., and Stange, H.H. 1954. *Deutsch. med. Wchnshr.* 79: 1519.
62. Plate, W.P. 1956. *Nederlands Tijdschrift voor Verlosk* 56: 37.
62a Plate, W.P. 1960. *Gynaecologia* 150: 267.
63. Rabinowitz, J.L., and Dowben, R.M. 1955. *Biochim. Biophys. Acta* 16: 96.
64. Rabinowitz, J.L., and Olekoyskyn, O. 1958. *Atomproaxi* 4: 85.
65. Rakoff, A.E. 1962. *J. Germantown Hosp.*, Feb., 25.
66. Ryan, K.J., and Smith, O.W. 1961. *J. Biol. Chem.* 236: 705.
67. Ryan, K.J., and Smith, O.W. 1961. *J. Biol. Chem.* 236: 2207.
68. Sandor, T., and Lanthier, A. 1960. *Rev. Canad. Biol.* 19: 445.
69. Savard, K., Gut, M., Dorfman, R.I., Gabrilove, J.L., and Soffer, L.J. 1961. *J. Clin. Endocrinol. & Metab.* 21: 165.
70. Seeman, A., and Saracino, R.T. 1961. *Acta Endocrinol.* 37: 31.
71. Segaloff, A., Gordon, D.L., Bowers, C.X., Schlosser, J.V., and Murison, P.H. 1957. *Cancer* 10: 1114.
72. Sendrail, M.L., Gleizes, L., Salvy-Sibloni, A.M. 1958. *Ann. Endocrinol.* 19: 824.
73. Sharma, D.C., Forchielli, E., and Dorfman, R.I. 1963, unpublished.
74. Shearman, R.P., Cox, R.I., and Gannon, A. 1961. *Lancet* 1: 260.
75. Short, R.V. 1960. *J. Endocrinol.* 20: 147.
76. Short, R.V. 1961. *Brit. Med. J.* 1: 1724.
77. Smith, O.W., and Ryan, K.J. 1961. *Endocrinology* 69: 869.
78. Solomen, S., Vande Wiele, R., and Lieberman, S. 1956. *J. Am. Chem. Soc.* 78: 5453.
79. Stein, I.F., and Leventhal, M.L. 1935. *Am. J. Obstet. & Gynecol.* 29: 181.
80. Stein, I.F., Cohen, M.R., and Elson, R. 1949. *Am. J. Obstet. & Gynecol.* 58: 267.

81. Sweat, M., Berliner, D., Bryson, M., Nabors, C., Jr., Haskell, S., and Holmstrom, E. 1960. *Biochim. Biophys. Acta* **40**: 289.
82. Tamaoki, B.I., and Pincus, G. 1961. *Endocrinology* **69**: 527.
83. Trace, R.J., Keaty, E.C., and McCall, M.L. 1960. *Am. J. Obstet. & Gynecol.* **79**: 310.
84. Warren, J.C., and Salhanick, A.A. 1961. *J. Clin. Endocrinol. & Metab.* **21**: 1218.
85. Wiest, W., Zander, G., and Holmstrom, E.G. 1959. *J. Clin. Endocrinol. & Metab.* **19**: 297.
86. Wilson, R.B., and Keating, F.R. 1958. *Am. J. Obstet. & Gynecol.* **76**: 388.
87. Wotiz, H.H., Davis, J.W., Lemon, H.M., and Gut, M. 1956. *J. Biol. Chem.* **222**: 487.
88. Zacco, M., Perrini, M., and D'Addabbo, A. 1956. *Folio Endocrinol.* **9**: 529.
89. Zander, J. 1958. *J. Biol. Chem.* **232**: 117.
90. Zenner, F.B. 1961. *Fertil. & Steril.* **12**: 25.

V

Virendra B. Mahesh, Ph.D., D.Phil, and
Robert B. Greenblatt, M.D., C.M.

SIGNIFICANCE OF EXCESSIVE ANDROGEN PRODUCTION BY THE POLYCYSTIC OVARY AND ITS RELATIONSHIP TO ENZYMATIC ABNORMALITIES

The role of the adrenals and the ovary as sources of androgens that cause hirsutism in the polycystic ovary syndrome has been a subject of much discussion in the past [5], [7], [16], [19], [23], [25], [35], [47], [48]. The observation of an increased excretion of "pregnane complex" and elevated levels of urinary pregn-5-ene-3β, 17α, 20α-triol in the polycystic ovary syndrome implicated the adrenals, as these compounds were hitherto known to be of pure adrenal origin [9], [16], [20]. Furthermore, the frequent finding of polycystic ovaries associated with androgen-secreting tumors of the adrenals, as well as in congenital adrenal hyperplasia, also suggested adrenal involvement in the polycystic ovary syndrome [13], [17], [28], [32], [33], [44], [48], [49].

The development of newer techniques and microchemical methods have enabled several investigators to re-evaluate the role of the ovary and the adrenals as a source of excessive androgens in the polycystic ovary syndrome. To obtain a comprehensive picture of the function of the polycystic ovaries under physiological conditions, Mahesh, et al. [37-43] have carried out the following studies in normal subjects and patients with the polycystic ovary syndrome:
1. urinary excretion of steroids before and after adrenal suppression and ovarian stimulation
2. steroid content of ovarian tissue
3. *in vitro* biosynthesis of steroids by the normal and polycystic ovary
4. steroid content of ovarian venous blood.

These studies have demonstrated that the polycystic ovary may be a potential source of androgens and the excessive androgen production may be associated with either a failure of aromatization of andros-4-ene-3, 17-dione to estrogens or the ovarian 3β-ol dehydrogenase. It is the purpose of this article to review the role of the ovaries as a source of androgens and their possible role in hirsutism.

60

SECRETION OF ANDROGENS BY NORMAL AND POLYCYSTIC OVARIES AS INDICATED BY URINARY STUDIES

Although mild androgenic properties were noted in ovarian extracts in 1925 by Champy and Kritch [8], the actual secretion of such compounds by the ovary was first suggested by the work of Dingemanse and Huis I'nt Veld in 1951 [10]. These investigators observed that there is a marked depression in urinary androsterone after castration in the female. The secretion of androgens by the polycystic ovary was first suggested by the work of Greenblatt in 1953 [22] who noted a decrease in urinary 17-ketosteroids in patients who had undergone wedge resection or panhysterectomy (Fig. 5-1). Such findings suggest the presence of 17-ketosteroid precursors of ovarian origin. Similar observations were made in regard to plasma dehydroepiandrosterone sulfate and androsterone sulfate after wedge resection of polycystic ovaries [26].

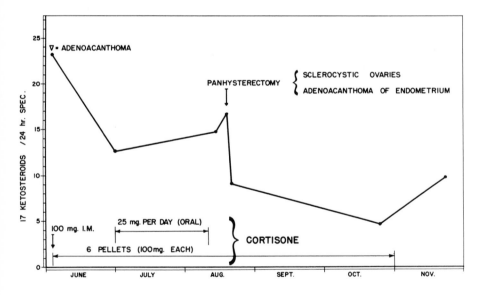

Fig. 5-1. Markedly Hirsute Female with Amenorrhea-Menorrhagia Syndrome*

The secretion of androgen by the normal and polycystic ovaries was studied by Mahesh and Greenblatt [40] by measuring urinary steroids before and after adrenal suppression and following stimulation of the ovaries with human pituitary FSH while the adrenals were kept suppressed. The results are presented in Table 5-1. In patients with polycystic ovaries, the levels of urinary dehydroepiandrosterone,

*Greenblatt [22]

androsterone and etiocholanolone, even after adrenal suppression, remained high as compared to those observed in women with normal ovaries. Moreover, there was a marked increase in the above-mentioned
steroids when human pituitary FSH was administered to patients with
the polycystic ovary syndrome, whereas in normal women there was
only a small elevation. The adrenals were kept under effective suppression during the FSH stimulation, as revealed by the study of
urinary tetrahydrocortico-steroids and 11-oxygenated-17-ketosteroids.
These findings indicate that the polycystic ovaries are capable of se-
creting large quantities of androgens. Poor depression of urinary 17-
ketosteroids after adrenal suppression in patients with Stein-Leventhal
syndrome has been reported also by other investigators [21], [25], [27].
An increase in urinary 17-ketosteroids after sheep and human pituitary
FSH administration has been observed by Keetal, et al. [30] and
Gemzell, et al. [18]. However, these investigators did not suppress
adrenal function prior to the administration of FSH, and therefore the
source of the 17-ketosteroid precursors was not completely established.

Table 5-1. Urinary Steroid Levels in MGM. per 24 Hr. in a Normal Patient
and One with Stein-Leventhal Syndrome Subjected to
Stimulating and Suppressive Measures*

Case No.	Patient with Stein-Leventhal syndrome	Dehydro-epiandrosterone	Etiocholanolone	Androsterone	Pregnanetriol	Pregn-5-ene-3β, 17α, 20α-triol	Tetrahydro-corticosteroids	11-Oxy-17-ketosteroids
IX	Control 1	<0.1	3.2	3.3	1.4	<0.1	9.1	1.1
	Control 2	<0.1	3.3	3.5	1.0	<0.1	9.3	1.3
	ACTH 1	1.0	5.5	5.9	1.8	1.5	37.7	5.2
	ACTH 2	1.4	5.9	6.4	2.8	2.9	39.2	5.7
	β-methasone 3	<0.1	1.9	2.1	0.8	<0.1	0.7	0.3
	β-methasone 4	<0.1	2.1	2.3	0.3	<0.1	0.4	<0.1
	FSH 5 (+ β-methasone)	0.5	7.4	6.1	3.2	8.8	<0.1	<0.1
	FSH 6 (+ β-methasone)	0.8	6.0	5.7	7.3	9.4	<0.1	<0.1
	Post-operative	<0.1	0.5	0.3	<0.1	<0.1	2.6	0.8
	Normal Subject							
IV	Control 1	0.2	2.1	0.9	0.4	0.2	4.0	2.1
	Control 2	0.1	2.2	0.7	0.3	0.2	4.2	1.8
	β-methasone 3	<0.1	0.7	0.3	<0.1	<0.1	0.4	0.1
	β-methasone 4	<0.1	0.4	0.2	<0.1	<0.1	0.3	<0.1
	FSH 5 (+ β-methasone)	<0.1	0.9	0.5	<0.1	<0.1	<0.1	<0.1
	FSH 6 (+ β-methasone)	<0.1	0.8	0.4	<0.1	<0.1	<0.1	<0.1

*Mahesh & Greenblatt [40]

STEROID CONTENT OF NORMAL AND POLYCYSTIC OVARIES

The steroid content of the tissues removed during wedge resection of the ovaries of normal women and patients with the polycystic ovary syndrome has been studied by Mahesh and Greenblatt [41]. Some of the patients under study did not receive any treatment, while others received human pituitary FSH prior to surgery. The findings in ten such cases are presented in Fig. 5-2.

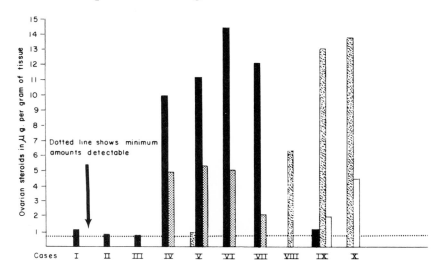

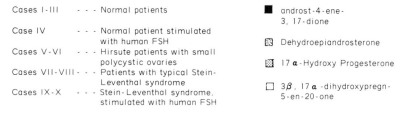

Cases I-III	- - - Normal patients	■ androst-4-ene-3, 17-dione
Case IV	- - - Normal patient stimulated with human FSH	
Cases V-VI	- - - Hirsute patients with small polycystic ovaries	▨ Dehydroepiandrosterone
Cases VII-VIII	- - - Patients with typical Stein-Leventhal syndrome	▨ 17 α -Hydroxy Progesterone
Cases IX-X	- - - Stein-Leventhal syndrome, stimulated with human FSH	□ 3β, 17 α -dihydroxypregn-5-en-20-one

Fig. 5-2. Steroid Content of Ovaries of Normal and Hirsute Female*

The normal ovary contained only small quantities of androst-4-ene-3, 17-dione (Cases I-III) and these results are in agreement with those of Zander [66]. The ovaries of patients with the polycystic ovary syndrome contained large quantities of either androst-4-ene-3, 17-dione and 17α-hydroxyprogesterone (Fig. 5-2, Cases V-VII) or dehydroepiandrosterone (Fig. 5-2, Case VIII). Furthermore, when such patients were treated with human pituitary FSH prior to surgery, the ovaries contained 17α-hydroxypregnenolone in addition to larger quantities of
*Mahesh and Greenblatt [43]

dehydroepiandrosterone (Fig. 5-2, Cases IX-X). Large quantities of androst-4-ene-3,17-dione have also been isolated from ovarian follicular fluid of patients with the Stein-Leventhal syndrome by Short and London [59]. However, these investigators did not find any dehydroepiandrosterone. It may be pertinent to mention that in our studies it was not possible to distinguish, histologically, polycystic ovaries that contained androst-4-ene-3,17-dione from those that contained dehydroepiandrosterone.

The formation of 17α-hydroxyprogesterone and androst-4-ene-3, 17-dione from progesterone in human and bovine ovaries has been shown by various investigators [2], [21], [29], [56], [60], [61], [62], [63]. Aromatization of androst-4-ene-3,17-dione or testosterone to estrogens has also been amply demonstrated [4], [65]. The *in vivo* conversion of 4-C^{14}-cholesterol to estrogens in the pregnant mare was reported by Heard and co-workers [24]. This conversion has been shown to occur also in the human ovary by Ryan and Smith [53]. From the results of these investigators, it is generally accepted that cholesterol is con-

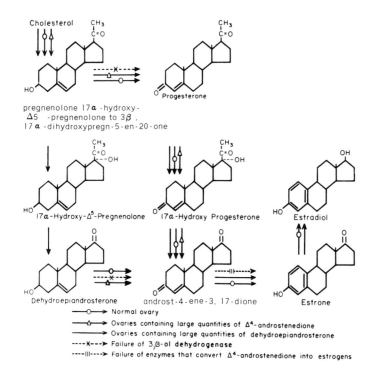

Fig. 5-3. Major Pathways of Biosynthesis of Steroids in the Ovary*

*Mahesh and Greenblatt [43]

verted into estrogens via pregnenolone, progesterone, 17α-hydroxy-progesterone and androst-4-ene-3, 17-dione (Fig. 5-3). The isolation of large quantities of 17α-hydroxyprogesterone and androst-4-ene-3, 17-dione from the ovary of a normal subject after *in vivo* stimulation with exogenous human pituitary FSH supports this pathway of biosynthesis (Fig. 5-2, Case IV).

The isolation of dehydroepiandrosterone from the polycystic ovaries of Stein-Leventhal syndrome (Fig. 5-2, Case VIII) and of 17α-hydroxypregnenolone with larger quantities of dehydroepiandrosterone (Fig. 5-2, Cases IX-X), following the *in vivo* stimulation of such ovaries with human pituitary FSH, indicates that dehydroepiandrosterone is probably synthesized from pregnenolone via 17α-hydroxypregnenolone (Fig. 5-3). The recent experiments of Ryan and Smith [54] suggest that this conversion takes place in the normal ovary as a minor route in the synthesis of estrogens from cholesterol.

STUDIES OF OVARIAN VENOUS BLOOD

"Free" Androgens

Seeman and Saracino [57] observed significantly higher levels of ketosteroids in ovarian venous blood as compared to peripheral blood in patients with the polycystic ovary syndrome. Mahesh and Greenblatt extracted free steroids from ovarian venous plasma and separated into testosterone, dehydroepiandrosterone, and androst-4-ene-3-17-dione fractions by paper chromatography [37]. The individual fractions were then converted into estrogens by incubation with a placental enzyme [52] and estimated by the method of Finkelstein, et al. [14]. The results are presented in Table 5-2. It is of interest to note the absence of detectable amounts of dehydroepiandrosterone, androst-4-ene-3, 17-dione, and testosterone in normal ovarian venous blood. However, when the normal ovary is stimulated with human pituitary FSH, small amounts of androst-4-ene-3, 17-dione are detectable. On the other hand, there are large quantities of androst-4-ene-3, 17-dione or dehydroepiandrosterone in both untreated and gonadotrophin-treated patients with Stein-Leventhal syndrome. Testosterone was not detectable in any of the ovarian venous blood studied. This study presents conclusive evidence for the secretion of abnormally large quantities of androgens by the polycystic ovary.

Estrogens

A study of the estrogen content of the ovarian venous blood was undertaken in normal subjects and patients with the polycystic ovary syndrome by the method of Preedy and Aitken [3], [51]. The results are also shown in Table 5-2. The concentration of estradiol in ovarian venous plasma of a normal female was 1.7 μg/100 ml around the time of ovulation. No estrone or estriol was detectable. When human pituitary FSH was administered to another normal female (Case IV), there was a marked increase in the level of estradiol. Patients with the polycystic ovary syndrome (Cases VI, VIII) secreted only small amounts of estradiol which were comparable to or less than that found in the venous blood of the normal ovary. Furthermore, no significant elevation was noted in estradiol content of ovarian venous blood of one such patient, even after stimulation with exogenous human pituitary FSH (Case IX).

Table 5-2.   Steroid Content of Ovarian Venous Blood from Normal and Polycystic Ovaries

Case No.	Vol. of ovarian venous plasma	Source of ovarian venous blood	Steroids in µg/100 ml of ovarian plasma			Estrogens in µg/100 ml of ovarian venous blood	
			Testosterone	Dehydroepi-androsterone	Androst-4-ene-3, 17-dione	Estradiol	Estrone or Estriol
IV	8 ml	Normal ovary - untreated	<0.4	<0.4	<0.4	1.7	<0.3
	3.8 ml	Normal ovary stimulated with HP-FSH	<0.7	<0.7	1.1	5.6	<0.6
VI	11 ml	Polycystic ovary - untreated	<0.3	<0.3	20.9	0.6	<0.2
VII	5.1 ml	Polycystic ovary - untreated	<0.5	<0.5	13.1		
VIII	6.2 ml	Polycystic ovary - untreated	<0.45	9.4	<0.45	1.1	<0.35
IX	5.4 ml	Polycystic ovary stimulated with HP-FSH	<0.5	15.4	<0.5	0.9	<0.4

SECRETION RATE STUDIES

The secretion rates of dehydroepiandrosterone and androst-4-ene-dione and testosterone* have been studied by MacDonald, Vande Wiele and Lieberman in normal women and patients with the Stein-Leventhal syndrome [36]. Their results also indicate increased rates of secretion of dehydroepiandrosterone or androst-4-enedione and testosterone in patients with Stein-Leventhal syndrome, even while the adrenals were suppressed.

Furthermore, ovarian suppression with estrogens depressed the androgen secretion to unmeasurable levels, while withdrawal of estrogen treatment restored the androgen secretion. These observations lend further support to the view that polycystic ovaries secrete androgens.

EVIDENCE INDICATING ENZYME DEFECTS IN THE POLYCYSTIC OVARY

It has been shown conclusively by the evidence presented above that the polycystic ovaries contain large quantities of androst-4-ene-3,17-dione or dehydroepiandrosterone and that these steroids are secreted by the ovaries. The normal ovary, on the other hand, contains only small quantities of androst-4-ene-3,17-dione, and very small amounts may be secreted. Furthermore, when the normal ovary is stimulated *in vivo* by exogenous human pituitary FSH, the synthesis of 17α-hydroxyprogesterone and androst-4-ene-3-17-dione is stepped up within the ovary (Case IV, Fig. 5-2), but these compounds may not be secreted by the ovary in any significant quantities, as shown by studies of ovarian venous blood and urinary steroids (Case IV, Tables 5-1 and 5-2). The *in vitro* biosynthesis of steroids in the normal and polycystic ovary has been studied by Mahesh and Green-blatt [38], and these investigations indicate two types of enzymatic abnormalities in the polycystic ovary.

ABNORMALITIES IN THE CONVERSION OF ANDROST-4-ENE-3,17-DIONE INTO ESTROGENS

Ovarian slices were incubated with 50 μg quantities of 4-C^{14}-androst-4-ene-3,17-dione and the estrogens thus formed were purified and estimated. The results are shown in Table 5-3. It is of interest

---

*As androst-4-ene-3,17-dione and testosterone give the same urinary metabolites, measurement of the total amount of these steroids was carried out. These studies do not give any indication whether polycystic ovaries secreted androst-4-ene-3,17-dione, testosterone, or both.

to note that the normal ovary (Case IV) and the polycystic ovaries that contained large quantities of dehydroepiandrosterone (Cases VIII-X) showed appreciable conversion of androst-4-ene-3,17-dione to estrogens, whereas the polycystic ovary that contained large quantities of androst-4-ene-3,17-dione (Case VI) showed only a very poor conversion of androst-4-ene-3,17-dione to estrogens. It should be pointed out that polycystic ovaries with high dehydroepiandrosterone content (Cases VIII-X) had abnormalities that led to the failure of synthesis of androst-4-ene-3,17-dione. However, when these ovaries were incubated with androst-4-ene-3,17-dione there was normal conversion of this substrate to estrogens. On the other hand, in the ovaries of Case VI, the abnormality lay in the aromatization of androst-4-ene-3, 17-dione to estrogens. The finding of larger quantities of androst-4-ene-3,17-dione in ovarian venous blood of Case VI as compared to that of normal subjects (Table 5-2) confirms this belief.

Table 5-3. Conversion of $7H^3$-dehydroepiandrosterone to androst-4-ene-3,17-dione and Conversion of $4C^{14}$ to Estrogens when 50 μg of the Precursors were Incubated with 1 g. Ovarian Slices

	Test for 3β-of dehydrogenase activity	Test for enzymes that convert androst-4-ene-3,17-dione into estrogens
	Incubation with $7H^3$-dehydroepiandrosterone-conversion to androst-4-ene-3,17-dione*	Incubation with $4C^{14}$-androst-4-ene-3,17-dione conversion to estrogens
Case IV normal	36.9 μg	26.1 μg
Case VI hirsute with slightly enlarged polycystic ovary	35.3 μg	3.2 μg
Case VIII Stein-Leventhal syndrome	4.7 μg	16.1 μg
Case IX Stein-Leventhal syndrome	4.6 μg	17.5 μg
Case X Stein-Leventhal syndrome	1.7 μg	21.4 μg

*This also includes conversion to estrogens.

This view is further supported by the observations of Short and London [59], who found large quantities of androst-4-ene-3,17-dione and no detectable amounts of estrogens in ovarian follicular fluid from patients with the Stein-Leventhal syndrome, in contrast to smaller quantities of androst-4-ene-3,17-dione along with appreciable amounts of estrogens in the ovarian follicular fluid of normal females. The *in vitro* studies of Axelrod and Goldzieher [2] also indicate such an enzymatic inadequacy.

ABNORMALITIES IN THE 3β-ol DEHYDROGENASE

In the generally accepted pathway of the biosynthesis of steroids in the normal ovary (Fig. 5-3), one of the major conversions is the transformation of pregnenolone to progesterone by the action of ovarian 3β-ol-dehydrogenase. The presence of large quantities of dehydroepiandrosterone in polycystic ovaries (Fig. 5-2, Cases VIII-X) seemed to indicate some abnormality in the 3β-ol-dehydrogenase. Ovarian slices were incubated with 7-H_3-dehydroepiandrosterone and the total conversion to androst-4-ene-3,17-dione and estrogens was measured (Table 5-3) [38]. The results showed that there was very poor 3β-ol dehydrogenase activity in polycystic ovaries that contained large quantities of dehydroepiandrosterone (Cases VIII-X) as compared to other ovaries studied (Cases IV, VI).

Such interpretation of the above observation is made on the assumption that the conversion of dehydroepiandrosterone to estrogens is mediated by the initial conversion of dehydroepiandrosterone to androst-4-ene-3, 17-dione by the action of the 3β-ol-dehydrogenase. The isolation of dehydroepiandrosterone in polycystic ovaries of untreated patients (Case VIII), and of larger quantities of dehydroepiandrosterone along with 17α-hydroxypregnenolone in the ovaries of patients with Stein-Leventhal syndrome after *in vivo* stimulation with exogenous human pituitary FSH, and the presence of dehydroepiandrosterone in ovarian venous blood in Cases VIII and IX (Table 5-2) all confirm the existence of abnormalities of 3β-ol dehydrogenase.

ESTROGEN SYNTHESIS AND EXCRETION IN THE POLYCYSTIC OVARY SYNDROME

Patients with the polycystic ovary syndrome consistently show moderate to good estrogen secretion as judged by breast development, vaginal smears and endometrial biopsies [23]. Several investigations on urinary estrogen levels in the polycystic ovary syndrome have been reported in the literature. In view of the unreliability of methods used, the earlier work will not be mentioned. The recent determinations of urinary estrogens in patients with the polycystic ovary syndrome using reliable methods have indicated that estrogen levels are within the limits of normal [6], [12], [50], [58]. Jayle, et al. [27] have reported higher average excretion of "phenolsteroids" in twenty patients with amenorrhea and virilism. However, no information is available on the state of the ovaries in this investigation.

Further light is thrown on this problem by the study of the steroid content of ovarian venous blood by Mahesh, et al. [43]. Even though the levels of estrogens in the ovarian venous blood from polycystic ovaries were comparable to that from the normal ovary, there were significant differences in the androgen-estrogen ratio in these cases. The differences in the ratios clearly demonstrate the presence of enzymatic abnormalities which result in a decrease in estrogen synthesis and an increase in androgen production. In view of the above observations, it may be argued that the finding of normal urinary excretion of estrogens does not rule out defective ovarian biosynthesis of estrogens.

Although it is clearly demonstrated by the above-mentioned studies that there are enzymatic abnormalities in the biosynthesis of estrogens in polycystic ovaries, nevertheless it is apparent that the block is not complete. The ovaries may still be able to produce physiological quantities of estrogens due to larger numbers of follicles participating in estrogen production. Furthermore, increased concentration of substrates present in ovarian tissue may also help to override the enzymatic block to some extent. In an attempt to produce physiological amounts of estradiol in the presence of enzymatic block, androgen synthesis is augmented. The *in vivo* metabolism of excessive androgens produced by the ovary to estrogens may be another factor that would contribute to estrogens in the urine. The *in vivo* conversion of androgens to estrogens has been demonstrated in normal women by Nathanson et al. [45] and in castrated and adrenalectomized human females by West, et al. [64].

ANDROGENS RESPONSIBLE FOR HIRSUTISM IN THE POLYCYSTIC OVARY SYNDROME

Dehydroepiandrosterone and androst-4-ene-3,17-dione have only weak androgenic activity in the human, and the question has been repeatedly raised whether they can account for the hirsutism in the polycystic ovary syndrome [29], [34], [56]. Conversion of radioactive progesterone and/or androst-4-ene-3,17-dione to testosterone has been reported in normal and polycystic ovaries and in tissue from an arrhenoblastoma by *in vitro* studies [15], [29], [55], [56], [63]. Likewise, the *in vitro* synthesis of testosterone from acetate-1-C^{14} has also been demonstrated in polycystic ovaries [34], [46]. Testosterone has been isolated from arrhenoblastoma tissue by Savard, et al. and Anliker, et al. [1], [56], and from the ovaries of a patient with hyperthecosis by Mahesh and Greenblatt [39]. These observations have led to the postulation that ovaries of patients with the polycystic ovary syndrome secrete testosterone. However, it is noteworthy that testosterone was not isolated from normal human ovarian tissue by Zander [66] or Mahesh, et al. [41], from human and bovine corpus luteum by Sweat, et al. [61], or from ovarian tissue and ovarian follicular fluid of patients with polycystic ovary syndrome by Mahesh, et al, [41] and Short, et al. [59]. Detectable quantities of testosterone were not present in ovarian venous blood of normal subjects and patients with the Stein-Leventhal syndrome [37].

Mahesh and Greenblatt have recently studied the plasma testosterone levels in normal women before and after oral administration of dehydroepiandrosterone and androst-4-ene-3,17-dione [42]. Their results clearly demonstrate the *in vivo* conversion of dehydroepiandrosterone and androst-4-ene-3,17-dione to testosterone in the human. This finding can explain the frequent occurrence of hirsutism in the polycystic ovary syndrome due to the conversion of the weaker androgens secreted by the ovary to a potent androgen, testosterone. The conversion of dehydroepiandrosterone to testosterone has been shown to occur in the liver [31]. It may also explain Dorfman's finding of elevated levels of plasma testosterone in hirsute females [11].

The authors wish to emphasize that although they have stressed the role of the ovary as a cause of hirsutism in the polycystic ovary syndrome, nevertheless there are cases in which the androgens from the adrenals are wholly or partly responsible for the hair growth. Furthermore, the polycystic ovary syndrome has many variants and our study is not broad enough so far to cover the entire spectrum of the syndrome. The studies during the past two years have contributed considerably to a better understanding of the problem. This field still has many untrodden territories that offer a challenge to future investigators.

SUMMARY

1. A study of the secretion of androgens by the normal and polycystic ovary has been carried out.

2. The normal ovary secretes only very small quantities of androgens as judged by steroid content of the ovary and urinary steroid studies before and after adrenal suppression.

3. The study of the steroid content of the polycystic ovary revealed two types of such ovaries. One of these types contained large quantities of anadrost-4-ene-3,17-dione and 17α-hydroxyprogesterone while the other contained dehydroepiandrosterone.

4. The levels of urinary dehydroepiandrosterone, androsterone, and etiocholanolone in patients with the polycystic ovary syndrome remain elevated even after adrenal suppression. This is in contrast to a marked depression noted in the levels of these urinary steroids in

normal females following such treatment. Furthermore, when the ovaries were stimulated with exogenous human pituitary FSH while the adrenals were kept suppressed, there was a marked rise in the above-mentioned steroids in the urine of patients with the Stein-Leventhal syndrome, whereas in normal subjects there was only a very small increase. The above-mentioned observations indicate the secretion of large amounts of androgens by the polycystic ovary.

5. Two types of ovarian enzymatic abnormalities were indicated by *in vitro* incubation of ovarian slices with $4C^{14}$-androst-4-ene-3,17-dione and $7-H^{3}$-dehydroepiandrosterone. They are (1) failure of aromatization of androst-4-ene-3,17-dione into estrogens and (2) failure of the 3β-ol-dehydrogenase.

6. The question has been raised repeatedly whether the secretion of weak androgens such as androst-4-ene-3,17-dione and dehydroepiandrosterone can account for the hirsutism in the polycystic ovary syndrome. The demonstration of the *in vivo* conversion of androst-4-ene-3,17-dione and dehydroepiandrosterone to testosterone in normal women makes it very tempting to postulate that the androgenic activity of these weak androgens is mediated by their conversion to testosterone.

REFERENCES

1. Anliker, R., Rohr, O., and Ruzicka, L. 1957. *Justus Liebigs Ann. Chem.* 603: 109.
2. Axelrod, L. R., and Goldzieher, J.W. 1961. *Arch. Biochem. Biophys.* 95: 547.
3. Aydar, C.K., Mahesh, V.B., and Greenblatt, R.B. Unpublished data.
4. Baggett, B., Engel, L.L., Savard, K., and Dorfman, R.I. 1956. *J. Biol. Chem.* 221: 931.
5. Brooks, R.V., and Prunty, F.T.G. 1960. *J. Endocrinol.* 21: 263.
6. Brown, J.B., and Matthew, G.D. 1962. *Rec. Prog. in Hormone Res.* 18: 337.
7. Buxton, C.L., and Vande Wiele, R. 1954. *New England J. Med.* 251: 293.
8. Champy, C., and Kritch, W. 1925. *Compt. Rend. Soc. Biol.* 92: 683.
9. Cox, R.I., and Shearman, R.P. 1961. *J. Clin. Endocrinol. & Metab.* 21: 586.
10. Dingemanse, E., and Hius In't Veld, L.G. 1951. *Acta Endocrinol.* 7: 71.
11. Dorfman, R.I. Personal communications.
12. Evans, T.N., and Riley, G.M. 1960. *Am. J. Obstet. & Gynec.* 80: 873.
13. Feher, L., Gyory, G., Less, E., and Laszlo, J. 1958. *Acta Endocrinol.* 28: 219.

14. Finkelstein, M., Forchielli, E., and Dorfman, R.I. 1961. *J. Clin. Endocrinol. & Metab.* 21: 98.
15. Forchielli, E., Gut, M., and Dorfman, R.I. 1961. *Proc. 43rd* Meeting Endocrine Soc., New York. Abstr. 46.
16. Gallagher, T.F., Kappas, A., Hellman, L., Lipsett, M.B., Pearson, O.H., and West, C.D. 1958. *J. Clin. Invest.* 37: 794.
17. Geist, S.H., and Gaines, J.A. 1942. *Am. J. Obstet. & Gynec.* 43: 975.
18. Gemzell, C.A., Dicsfalusy, E., and Tillinger, K.G. 1958. *J. Clin. Endocrinol. & Metab.* 18: 1333.
19. Gemzell, C.A., Tillinger, K.G., and Westman, A. 1959. *Acta Endocrinol.* 30: 387.
20. Gold, J.J., and Frank, R. 1958. *Am. J. Obstet. & Gynec.* 75: 1034.
21. Goldzieher, J.W., and Axelrod, L.R. 1960. *Acta Endocrinol.* 35 Suppl. 51: 617.
22. Greenblatt, R.B. 1953. *Am. J. Obstet. & Gynec.* 66: 700.
23. Greenblatt, R.B., and Baldwin, K.R. 1960. *Clin. Endocrinol.* 1, 498 (Grune & Stratton, Inc.)
24. Heard, R.D.H., Bligh, E.G., Cann, M.C., Jellinck, P.H., O'Donnell, V.J., Rao, B.G., and Webb, J.L. 1956. *Rec. Prog. in Hormone Res.* 12: 45.
25. Herrmann, W., Buckner, F., and Morris, J. McL. 1960. *Fertil. & Steril.* 11: 74.
26. Herrmann, W., Conrad, S.H., and Mahesh, V.B. 1961. *Proc. 43rd Meeting Endocrine Soc.*, New York. 1961. Abstr. 127: 67.
27. Jayle, M.F., Scholler, R., Mauvais-Jarvis, P., and Metay, S. 1961. *Acta Endocrinol.* 36: 375.
28. Jones, H.W., and Jones, G.E.S. 1954. *Am. J. Obstet. & Gynec.* 68: 1330.
29. Kase, N., Forchielli, E., and Dorfman, R.I. 1961. *Acta Endocrinol.* 37: 19.
30. Keettel, W.C., Bradbury, J.T., and Stoddard, F.J. 1957. *Am. J. Obstet. & Gynec.* 73: 954.
31. Klempien, E.J., Voigt, K.D., and Tamm, J. 1961. *Acta Endocrinol.* 36: 498.
32. Kovacic, N. 1959. *J. Clin. Endocrinol. & Metab.* 19: 844.
33. Landing, B.H. 1954. *J. Clin. Endocrinol. & Metab.* 14: 245.
34. Leon, N., Castro, M.N., and Dorfman, R.I. 1962. *Acta Endocrinol.* 39: 411.
35. Lipsett, M.B., and Riter, B. 1960. *J. Clin. Endocrinol. & Metab.* 20: 180.
36. MacDonald, P., Vande Wiele, R., and Lieberman, S. 1963. *Am. J. Obstet. & Gynec.* 86: 1.
37. Mahesh, V.B., Aydar, C.K., and Greenblatt, R.B. Unpublished data.

38. Mahesh, V. B., and Greenblatt, R. B. Unpublished data.
39. Mahesh, V. B., and Greenblatt, R. B. 1961. *Proc. 43rd Meeting Endocrine Soc.*, New York. Abstr. 151: 80.
40. Mahesh, V. B., and Greenblatt, R. B. 1961. *Nature* 191: 888.
41. Mahesh, V. B., and Greenblatt, R. B. 1962. *J. Clin. Endocrinol. & Metab.* 22: 441.
42. Mahesh, V. B., and Greenblatt, R. B. 1962. *Acta Endocrinol.* 41: 400.
43. Mahesh, V. B., Greenblatt, R. B., Aydar, C. K., and Roy, S. 1962. *Fertil. & Steril.* 13: 513.
44. Milcou, S. M., Pitis, M., Stanesco, V., Serban, A., Leiba, S., Nedelniuc, E., and Opran, H. 1960. *Sem. Hop. Paris.* 36: 1144.
45. Nathanson, I. T., Engel, L. L., and Kelley, R. M. 1952. *J. Clin. Endocrinol. & Metab.* 12: 1172.
46. O'Donnell, V., and McCaig, J. 1959. *Biochemical J.* 71: 9P.
47. Perloff, W. H., Hadd, H. E., Channick, B. J., and Nodine, J. H. 1957. *Arch. Int. Medic.* 100: 981.
48. Perloff, W. H., Channick, B. J., Suplick, B., and Carrington, E. R. 1958. *J. A. M. A.* 167: 2041.
49. Perloff, W. H., Channick, B. J., Hadd, H. E., and Nodine, J. H. 1958. *Fertil. & Steril.* 9: 247.
50. Preedy, J. R. K. Personal communications.
51. Preedy, J. R. K., and Aitken, E. H. 1961. *J. Biol. Chem.* 236: 1300.
52. Ryan, K. J. 1959. *J. Biol. Chem.* 234: 268.
53. Ryan, K. J., and Smith, O. W. 1961. *J. Biol. Chem.* 236: 2204.
54. Ryan, K. J., and Smith, O. W. 1961. *J. Biol. Chem.* 236: 2207.
55. Sandor, T., and Lanthier, A. 1960. *Rev. Canad. Biol.* 19: 445.
56. Savard, K., Gut, M., Dorfman, R. I., Gabrilov, J. L., and Soffer, L. J. 1961. *J. Clin. Endocrinol. & Metab.* 21: 165.
57. Seeman, A., and Saracino, R. T. 1961. *Acta Endocrinol.* 37: 31.
58. Shearman, R. P., Cox, R. I., and Gannon A. 1961. *Lancet* 1: 260.
59. Short, R. V., and London, D. R. 1961. *Brit. Med. J.* 1: 1724.
60. Solomon, S. S., Vande Wiele, R., and Lieberman, S. 1956. *J. Am. Chem. Soc.* 78: 5453.
61. Sweat, N. L., Berliner, D. L., Bryson, M. J., Nabors, C., Haskell, J., and Holmstrom, E. C. 1960. *Biochim. Biophys. Acta.* 40: 289.
62. Warren, J. C., and Salhanick, H. A. 1961. *J. Clin. Endocrinol. & Metab.* 21: 1218.
63. Wiest, W. C., Zander, J., and Holmstrom, E. G. 1959. *J. Clin. Endocrinol. & Metab.* 19: 297.
64. West, C. D., Damast, B. L., Sarro, S. D., and Pearson, O. H. 1956. *J. Biol. Chem.* 218: 409.
65. Wotiz, H. H., Davis, J. W., Lemon, H. M., and Gut, M. 1956. *J. Biol. Chem.* 222: 487.
66. Zander, J. 1958. *J. Biol. Chem.* 232: 117.

VI

Manuel Neves e Castro, M.D.
J. Neves Da Silva, M.D., and A. Reis Valle, M.D.

OVARIAN VIRILIZING SYNDROMES

In the past, especially when dealing with Latin races, and prior to the advent of new techniques for the assay of androgens, most cases of hirsutism were diagnosed as idiopathic, since no apparent etiologic factors could be easily detected. The physician was then faced with a considerably high incidence of hirsute women with no other symptoms or signs other than those of menstrual irregularities.

The recognition of adrenal cortical hyperfunction syndromes and of the co-existence of polycystic ovaries [24] with hirsutism opened new fields for the investigation of this abnormality of body hair growth in those patients with no apparent pathology.

The purpose of the present paper is to report on some of our patients with the ovarian virilizing syndrome. The following assays have been employed: urinary gonadotropins (HPG) [14], 17-ketosteroids (17-KS) [27], 17-ketogenic steroids (17-KGS) [1], estrogens [4], pregnanediol [13], and pregnanetriol [6], [7].

CASE NO. 1: (#192.931)

M.J.N.P. - White female, age 16, weighing 56.6 kg, height 1.48 m who came to the endocrine out-patient clinic of the Portugese Cancer Institute in April, 1961. She had had her menarche at the age of 9 and menstruated regularly every 28 days, with an 8-day flow. She had some degree of dysmenorrhea and occasional premenstrual tension. Soon after her menarche she noticed a gradual onset of hirsutism, mainly around the nipples and the umbilical-pubic lines, and later on the arms, thighs, legs, chin, and face. Her breasts had a perfectly normal development and never showed any volume decrease. Her body configuration has always been feminine. At the age of 14 she became amenorrheic. However, in January 1962 she resumed menstruation; from then on it has been quite scanty and the patient has had irregular and long cycles. The patient shaved daily. Psychologically, this girl has felt a progressively increasing sex drive. This, in fact, led her into prostitution, and even while at the hospital she tried to have homosexual contacts. There is no family history of hirsutism. On physical examination, aside from the general body appearance and hirsutism (Figs. 6-1 and 6-2), no abnormal signs were found except a very small uterus. The ovaries could hardly be palpated. There

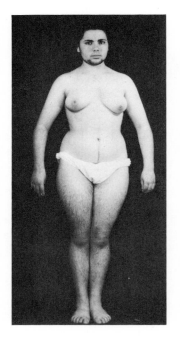
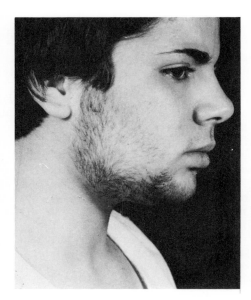

Fig. 6-1. M. J. N. P. – White female.   Fig. 6-2. M. J. N. P. – White female.
Age 16. (#192.931)   Age 16. (#192.931)

was slight clitoral hypertrophy (Fig. 6-3). She had a pneumorecto-peritoneum done and serial tomographies for visualization of the adrenals (Figs. 6-4, 6-5, and 6-6). The adrenals were found to be normal, and on the left side a round shadow was seen which was interpreted by some as the spleen and by others as a tumor. An I. V. pyelogram followed; no abnormalities were seen (Fig. 6-6).

Laboratory Findings:

Blood pressure: 130/100 mm Hg. Some of the more important laboratory studies are mentioned below.

Blood chemistry: Cholesterol (total) - 311 mg/100 ml; cholesterol esters - 128 mg/100 ml; alkaline phosphatase - 3.48 Bodansky units/100 ml; acid phosphatase 1.80 Bodansky units/100 ml; N. P. nitrogen - 20 mg/100 ml; sodium 143.4 mEq/L; potassium - 4.4 mEq/L.

Glucose tolerance test: fasting level - 97.5 mg/100 ml. After the ingestion of glucose solution: at 30 minutes - 147.5 mg/100 ml; at 60 minutes - 153 mg/100 ml; at 120 minutes - 132.5 mg/100 ml. There was no glycosuria.

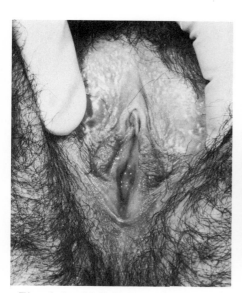

Fig. 6-3. M. J. N. P. - (#192.931) -
Moderate Hypertrophy
of the Clitoris

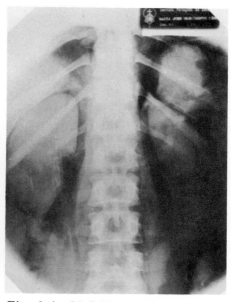

Fig. 6-4. M. J. N. P. - (#192.931) -
Pneumorectoperitoneum.
Flat Film

Electrophoresis of serum proteins: (Total proteins: 7.3 gm/100 ml). Albumin - 35.4 per cent; α_1 globulin - 4.9 per cent; α_2 globulin - 12.0 per cent; β globulin - 20.8 per cent; α globulin - 26.9 per cent.

Blood cytology: 3,680,000; 7,000 (hemoglobin 76 per cent). Thyroidal I_{131} uptake - 30 per cent after six hours and 55 per cent after 24 hours B. M. R. = + 13 per cent.

Electroencephalogram: normal.

Funduscopy: normal.

Radiography of the skull: no abnormalities noted.

Urine analysis: normal.

Hormonal studies: The initial values of the urinary assays were: 17-ketosteroids - 23.2 mg/24 hours; 17-ketogenic steroids - 15.5 mg/24 hours; Pregnanediol - 2.2 mg/24 hours; Estrone - 4 μg/24 hours; Estradiol-17β - 0; Estriol - 6.4 μg/24 hours.

The results of the suppression test with dexamethasone and a stimulation with corticotropin ACTH are shown in Fig. 6-7.

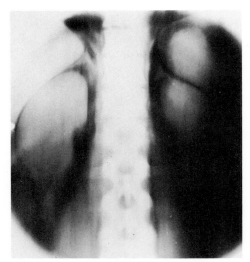

Fig. 6-5. M. J. N. P. - (#192.931) - Pneumorectoperitoneum
Tomogram (7 cm)

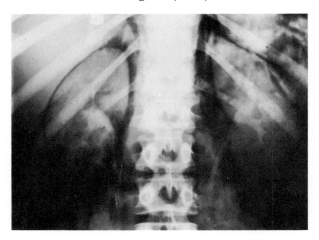

Fig. 6-6. M. J. N. P. - (#192.931) - I. V. Pyelogram 5 mn Following
the Injection of the Contrast

We were fortunate to determine the testosterone plasma levels of this patient. (See Chapter 2.) The initial values were 0.62 μg/100 ml of plasma (normal range for women 0.02-0.26 μg/100 ml of plasma).

In view of the sensitivity of the 17-KS and 17-KGS levels to dexamethasone and ACTH, and considering the equivocal results of the pneumorectoperitoneum, it was decided to explore the adrenals first.

The patient had an exploratory incision done in the left hypochondrium to expose the left adrenal. It was found that: (1) the adrenal cortex was markedly atrophied, (2) no tumor could be found, (3) in a palpatation through the peritoneal cavity the right adrenal was normal size, and (4) the shade seen in the X ray over the left kidney corresponded to the spleen. An infra-umbilical laparotomy was then done and the ovaries visualized. These were normal in size and white. A wedge resecection of both ovaries was performed; there was marked thickening of the capsule and many small cysts of a similar volume in a single row, underlying the thickened capsule. The uterus was very small. There were no other abnormalities. The wedges from these ovaries are being studied by incubation methods to clarify the steroid biosynthesis.

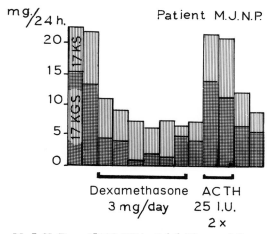

Fig. 6-7. M. J. N. P. - (#192.931) - Inhibition and Suppression Tests

Following operation the testosterone plasma levels decreased to 0.22 µg/100 ml (which is within the normal range for women). Other postoperative values were as follows: 17-KS - 14.3 mg/hours; 17-KGS - 12.8 mg/24 hours; Estrone - -4.8 µg/24 hours; Estradiol-17β - 5.3 µg/24 hours; Estriol - -6.7 µg/24 hours; Dehydroepiandrosterone - 0.94 mg/24 hours; Pregnanediol - 2.3 mg/24 hours.

This patient started having entirely normal monthly menstrual periods and biphasic basal body temperature charts, and has continued to up to the present time (August, 1962). One year after operation she still shaves, but less frequently. There seems to be a slight decrease of the hair growth.

PATHOLOGY REPORT

A fragment of the right ovary was received at the Department of Pathology (May 4, 1961) (No. 150.130) The preoperative diagnosis was: hirsutism, Stein-Leventhal syndrome?

Gross Appearance: Fragment of an ovary with the approximate size of a small bean. One of its faces was regular and smooth, corresponding to the cortex. Underlying this layer there were small cysts, some of them already opened, and others still preserved and filled with a clear fluid.

Microscopic Study: Multiple sections were made perpendicular to the cortical layer in order to study all cysts. The stains used in this study were: Hemalumen-Eosin, Van Gieson's, Masson's trichromic, and Tibor Papp's.

To the periphery a slightly thickened and fibrous tunica albuginea could be seen over numerous primordial follicles. The cysts were follicular in type, sometimes crumpled, outlined by several layers of cubic cells of variable thickness. This layer of granulosa cells of the follicular cysts was thinner whenever associated with the changes of the theca interna mentioned below (Fig. 6-8).

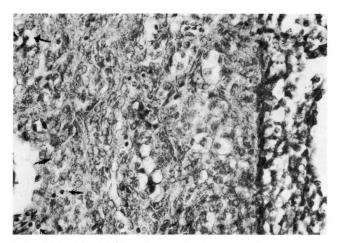

Fig. 6-8. No. 150.130/61. H. Eos. 350x. - Marked hyperthecosis. Theca externa: slight luteinization, hypochromatic cells, odema. Stroma lutein cells (to the left, see arrows)

There was hypertrophy of the theca interna due to hyperplasia of the cells (theca - lutein cells) which underwent luteinization. The nuclei were hyperchromatic and several mitotic figures were seen as well as an increased vascularization. The theca externa was slightly luteinized. The cells were hyperchromatic and edema was present. * In the same field (Fig. 6-8) small groups of stroma luteinized cells

---

*These changes are known as hyperthecosis. Sometimes it is accompanied by luteinization of the theca externa. This layer may, nevertheless, show only edema. The cells become less chromatic and may look more like epithelioid cells in contrast with their usual staining characteristics of stromal cells.

could be seen. The limiting membrane was always demonstrable particularly in the silver stained sections. In all sections, neither corpora lutea, corpora fibrosa, nor corpora albicantes were demonstrable.*
Comment: Although it was not possible to study both ovaries, the morphologic pattern of this fragment of an ovary is compatible with the diagnosis of Stein-Leventhal syndrome [2], [3], [5], [8-12], [15-26].

CASE NO. II (#198.702)

B. R. C. - White female, age 28 years, weighing 78 kg; height 1.60 m. The main complaint was periods of amenorrhea lasting from three to six months, since the age of menarch (age 11 years). The menses were very scanty. The patient stated that during the last years the intervals between menses have been progressively increasing. Primary infertility, weight increase, and hirsutism were noted.

Physical examination:

The main features were obesity with no pecularities and no striae. Moderate hirsutism was noted on the chin, lips, breasts, umbilico-pubic line, arms and forearms, thighs and legs. The pelvic examination did not disclose any abnormalities except slightly enlarged (?) and painful ovaries. There was no hypertrophy of the clitoris.
Blood pressure: 135/95 mm Hg.
Blood chemistry: Cholesterol (total) - 267 mg/100 ml; sodium 152 mEq/L; potassium 4.4 mEq/L; N. P. nitrogen - 0.34 gm/L
Glucose tolerance test: Fasting level - 120 mg/100 ml; 30 mn - 123 mg/100 ml; 60 mn 130 mg/100 ml; 120 mn - 103 mg/100 ml. No glycosuria.
Blood cytology: RBC. - 3,960,000; WBC. 7,200; hemoglobin 80 per cent.
Urine analysis: normal.
Endometrial biopsy: moderate cystic hyperplasia. No signs of secretory activity.
Hormone assays: 17 KS - 7.4 mg/24 hours; 17 KGS - 12.1 mg/24 hours; Estrone - -16.1 μg/24 hours; Estriol - 32 μg/24 hours.
In view of the symptomatology and hormone assays it was decided to perform an exploratory laparotomy. This revealed a normal-sized uterus and enlarged, pale, hard ovaries. A wedge resection was done on both ovaries. Following surgery the patient started having normal ovulatory menstrual cycles and noticed a decrease of the hirsutism. The post-operative level of 17 KS is 7.2 mg/24 hours and the 17 KGS-9.9 mg/24 hours.

---

*This may not be significant due to the small size of this fragment of tissue. Most of the ressected ovarian wedge was used for in vitro tissue incubation studies.

PATHOLOGY REPORT

April 3, 1962. Two wedges resected from the right ovary (No. 3103/62) and the left ovary (No. 3104/62) were received for microscopic examination. The clinical diagnosis was hirsutism, Stein-Leventhal syndrome (?). Since both the gross appearance and histological changes of these fragments are quite different, they will be separately described.

Left Ovary

Gross Appearance: This was an elongated, irregular fragment measuring 6 × 4 cm. It had a round, pale face (cortical) and a concave, slightly granular, brown red face which corresponded to an opened cyst. In parallel cross sections, perpendicular to the length of the fragment, one could see that the cavity was outlined by a thin superficial outer layer of ovarian stroma, followed by a generally thickened middle layer, yellow-brownish, and finally by a dark brown, thin inner layer. (Fig. 6-9). Close to one of the ends of the fragment, surrounded by a denser stroma, there was a small cyst, about the size of a pea, filled with a clear fluid.

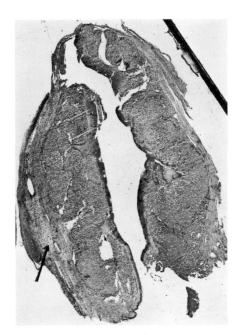

Fig. 6-9. No. 3103/62. H. Eos. 7x. - Left ovary: outer layer of ovarian stroma. To the left (arrows) paralutein cells. Medial layer of thick lutein cells. Inner layer which outlines the cavity.

Microscopic Study: The middle layer of the wall of the cyst was formed by large lutein cells, often with spongy cytoplasm; some of these cells showed one single large vacuole and picnotic nuclei. In other fields, stroma luteinization could be seen, i.e., paraluteinization, as well as many dilated blood vessels (Fig. 6-10). Paraluteinization was also observable as islets separated from the lutein layer. The internal layer of the cavity showed fibrin, fibroblasts, and hemosiderophages. The surface of the fragment corresponded to a slightly fibrous ovarian stroma. The wall of the small cyst showed a slight hypertrophy and luteinization of the theca interna. No signs of ovarian stroma hyperplasia could be seen.

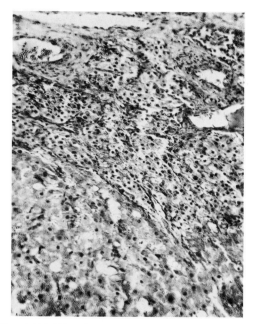

Fig. 6-10. No. 3103/62. H. Eos. 138x. - Left ovary: detail of the wall of the cyst. To the left, lutein cells in regression. To the right, paralutein cells and blood vessels.

Right Ovary

Gross Appearance: Wedge measuring 5 x 2 cm. The free surface was pale, round, and smooth, showing small mounds. The tunica albuginea was very thickened and fibrous. Underneath, there were numerous small cysts of different sizes, in the cortical, as a crown. In the central zone there were a few scars resembling corpora albicans (Fig. 6-11) and small clearer areas, which probably corresponded to stromal hyperplasia.

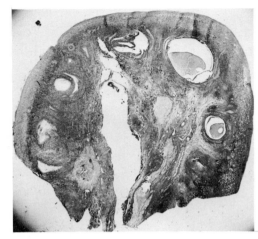

Fig. 6-11. No. 3104/62. H. Eos. 5x. - Right ovary: thick tunica albuginea. In the cortical, several cysts of variable size, as in a crown. Few scars. Slight stromal hyperplasia.

Microscopy Study: This showed that the cysts were follicular in type, some of them with hyperthecosis. In some areas, as the one in Fig. 6-12, there were hyperchromatic nuclei, many mitoses, luteinization, and pronounced vascularization. This resulted in a sharp hypertrophy of the theca interna, i. e., hyperthecosis. However, the granulosa cell

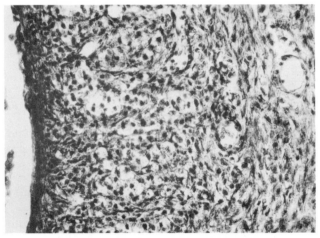

Fig. 6-12. No. 3104/62. H. Eos. 265x. - Right ovary: very pronounced hyperthecosis, hyperchromatism, mitosis, capillaries. The granulosa cell layer is thin and poorly preserved. Theca externa: edema, hypochromatism and scanty luteinization.

layer was not very prominent. There were rare paralutein cells in the theca externa, which in turn showed edema and a low affinity for the stains. There were no stroma lutein cells. Ovarian stroma hyperplasia could only be suspected in very small areas.

Comment: These observations suggest the diagnosis of Stein-Leventhal syndrome. There were a corpus luteum cyst and small islets of stromal luteinization in the left ovary [2], [3], [5], [8-12], [15-26].

CASE No. III: (#204.938)

M. M. F. - White female, age 28, weighing 45.1 kg. Height: 1.43 m. Eight years ago she noticed the onset of hirsutism which became more evident during the last two years. Simultaneously, and for the last two years, she complained of hypogastric pains. The pain, which was first paroxysmal in type, is now constant, and radiates to the left lumbar region. Movements of the left thigh tend to increase the pain. The pitch of the voice and libido are unchanged, but significant weight loss occurred. Breasts have not shown volume changes. From the age of the menarche (17 years of age) up to two years ago, she had normal monthly menses. From then on she has had oligomenorrhea and scanty flow. She shows primary infertility. She also experiences hypogastric pain on micturition.

Physical examination:

This revealed marked hirsutism (Figs. 6-13, 6-14, 6-15, and 6-16) and well-developed breasts (Fig. 6-17). Abdominal palpation was very painful in the hypogastrium, which interfered with observation of possible abdominal tumors. The liver and spleen were not palpable. The clitoris was hypertrophied. The pelvic examination was very painful. The uterus was smooth and the left adnexa seemed to be hard and enlarged.

Blood chemistry: Cholesterol (total) - 216.5 mg per cent; N. P. nitrogen - 0.32 gm/L; fasting blood sugar - 93 mg/100 ml; sodium - 123.9 mEq/L; potassium - 5.2 mEq/L.

Blood cytology: 3,700.000; 8,800. Hemoglobin 80 per cent.

Hormone assays: 17 KS - 11.2 mg/24 hours; 17 KGS - 15.4 mg/24 hours. An I. V. perfusion of 25 mg of prednisolone for an eight-hour period, with urine collected in the eight-hour period preceding and following the infusion, showed a good suppression of the 17 KS from 3.45 mg/8 hours to 1.80 mg/8 hours, and of the 17 KGS from 8.26 mg/8 hours to 3.20 mg/8 hours. Stimulation with 25 I. U. of corticotropin ACTH perfused over an eight-hour period on two successive days showed almost no change of the 17 KS (11.2 mg/24 hours to 12.53 mg/24 hours) and an elevation of the 17 KGS from 15.4 mg/24 hours to 25.8 mg/24 hours.

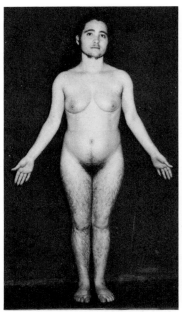

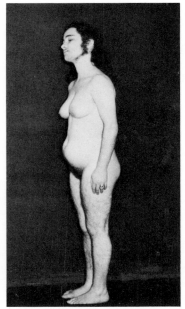

Fig. 6-13. M. M. F. – White female.
Age 28. (#204.938).

Fig. 6-14. M. M. F. – White female.
Age 28. (#204.938).

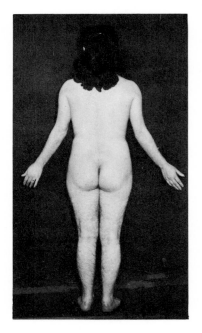

Fig. 6-15. M. M. F. – White female.
Age 28. (#204.938)

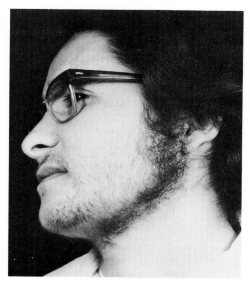

Fig. 6-16. M.M.F. - White female. Age 28. (#204.938)

In view of the suspicion of malignancy, immediate surgery was performed. Although there were doubts as to the nature of the tumor found, this tumor was removed.

Following the operation the patient received radioactive gold in the abdominal cavity and later had cobalt therapy. After the second operation the 17 KS - 4.3 mg/24 hours and the 17 KGS - 3.3 mg/24 hours.

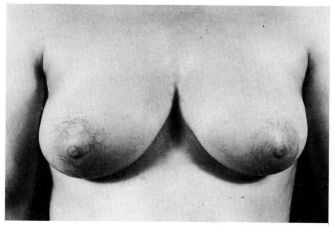

Fig. 6-17. M.M.F. - White female. Age 28. (#204.938).
Hypertrichosis around the nipples.

PATHOLOGY REPORT

The clinical diagnosis was: virilizing tumor of the ovary. Malignancy? The patient was operated on February 27, 1962 and the left adnexa and a wedge resected from the right ovary were sent to the Department of Pathology (No. 1982/62).

Gross Appearance: *Wedge from the right ovary* - This fragment, wedge-shaped, showed on its pale surface two pink papillary outgrowths; around them the surface was smooth and through it could be seen several cysts. In the cross sections many cysts filled with clear, sometimes cloudy, fluid were seen. Most of these cysts were small, the larger being the size of a pea. One of these cysts was filled up with pink wart-like papillary ingrowths which seemed to be connected with the superficial ones. In the stroma there were a few scars and smaller darker spots. The tunica albuginea was normal. In the cortex there were a few primordial follicles. *Left adnexa* - The tube was thick and sinuous. Its serosa coat was irregular and had adherences to the ovary. Its lumen was wider than the usual and the endosalpinx was thickened. The infundibulum showed adhered fimbriae. The ovary, spheroid in shape, was slightly enlarged, measuring 5 cm in diameter. There was a small papillary outgrowth (Fig. 6-18) similar to the one seen in the right ovary, which had a very thin pedicle. The surface of the ovary

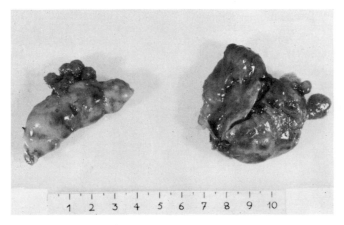

Fig. 6-18. - No. 1982/62. Right ovary: wedge with papillary outgrowth and irregularity of the surface due to the underlying cysts. Left adnexa: ovary enlarged. Papillary vegetations to the right. Surface irregularities due to cysts. To the left, tube can be seen.

was white and pale and showed several irregularities which corresponded to the underlying cysts. There were many cysts, most of them opened. However, the larger one had its lumen completely filled up with soft, pink papillary growths (Fig. 6-19). The other cysts contained a clear and sometimes colored fluid, lying under the albuginea like a crown. This tunica was thick and fibrous (Figs. 6-19 and 6-20). There were some scars in the inner portions of the ovary and small dark spots scattered in larger and lighter areas of fibrosis.

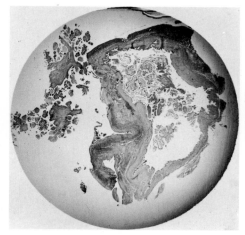

Fig. 6-19. No. 1982/62. H. Eos. 5x. - Left ovary: exophytic formation and papillary growths within the larger cyst. Thick albuginea.

Microscopic Study: This was entirely similar in all sections in so far as the papillary growths were concerned. There was a typical papillary structure with exophitic growth (Figs. 6-19 and 6-21). The continuity of the external portion of the tumor with the intracystic one could be seen and was due to rupture of the wall of the cyst (Fig. 6-21). The histologic pattern was the same in the intracystic and in the external growth of this tumor. Within the vegetations gland-like cavities

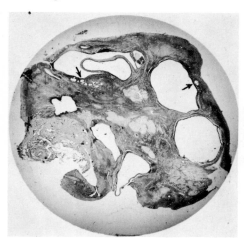

Fig. 6-20. No. 1982/62. H. Eos. 3.5x. - Left ovary: multiple cysts in the cortical. Thick albuginea. Some scars. Minimal areas of stromal hyperplasia. Small intracystic papillomas (arrows). To the lower left: hilus and blood vessels.

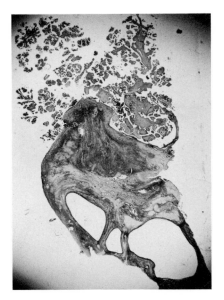

Fig. 6-21. No. 1982/62. H. Eos. 5x.
- Right ovary: continuity of the intracystic with the extracystic portion of
the tumor. Several cysts. Slightly
thickened albuginea. Some scars. In
the upper part, stromal hyperplasia.

were present. The vegetations and these cavities were lined by a cy-
lindrical, cubic epithelium of tubular type, in several layers, irregular,
with no order or polarity (Fig. 6-22). One could therefore see a
stratified epithelium, with hyperchromatic nuclei, and many mitotic
figures besides the invasion of the stroma. Some stroma were rich in

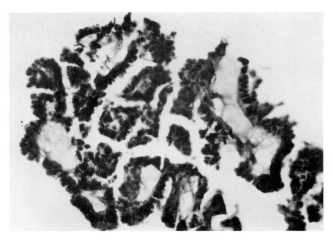

Fig. 6-22. No. 1982/62. H. Eos. 265x. - Right ovary: small
vegetations. Irregularly stratified epithelium. Hyperchromatism
and anisocariosis. Mitosis. Gelatinous and thin axes of the villi.

fibroblasts, and others are fibrous and hyalinized, showing numerous calcifications, which were typical psammoma bodies. Under the serosa of the left tube and on the surface of both ovaries there were numerous malignant granules. These were small cavities outlined by the described malignant epithelium and enveloped by connective tissue with many blood vessels and small round cells. The psammoma bodies were very abundant in the tubal lesions. Many of the walls of the cysts in both ovaries had marked hyperthecosis (Figs. 6-23 and 6-24). There was, as well, a fibrous thickening of the tunica albuginea. Several scars of corpora fibrosa and corpora albicantes were seen. There was ovarian stroma hyperplasia.

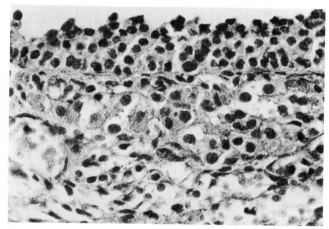

Fig. 6-23. No. 1982/62. H. Eos. 574x. - Theca interna: pronounded luteinization, hyperchromatism, mitosis and blood capillaries.

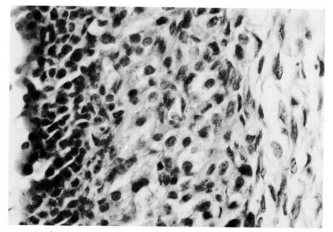

Fig. 6-24. No. 1982/62. H. Eos. 574x. - Right ovary (first operation): marked hyperthecosis. Theca externa; no luteinization, edema and poorly stained cells.

Comment: This is a bilateral papillary serous adenocarcinoma of the ovary with extensions into the peritoneal serosa. This malignancy arises from polycystic ovaries with hyperthecosis.

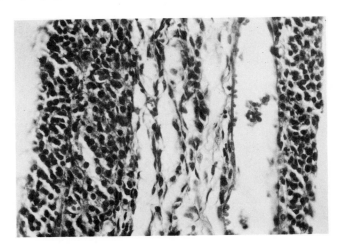

Fig. 6-25. No. 2477/62. H. Eos. 353x. - Right ovary (second operation): septum between two cysts. In the left, moderate hyperthecosis and edema of the theca externa. To the right, granulosa cell layer and a blood vessel; the theca is not luteinized and continues to the left one.

March 14, 1962. Total hysterectomy, unilateral oöphorectomy and omentectomy (Nos. 2476/62 and 2477/62).

Gross Appearance: *Uterus* - The cervix was normal. The corpus was normal in shape and in size (Fig. 6-26). However, its serosa was thick and irregular, and had yellow granules all over its surface. These granules were larger, more abundant, and confluent around the fundus and the posterior side. The miometrium was hard and slightly thickened. The endometrium was smooth and thin. *Right adnexa* - The tube was thick and straight. The serosa was not brilliant and had adhesions to the ovary. The ovary was irregular and still showed suture stitches from the previous operation. The lumen of the tube was increased and was filled with the folds of the mucosa, which appeared larger than usual. In the serosa and on the surface of the ovary there were yellow-bloody granules which were larger where the tube was attached to the ovary. *Ovary* - In the cross sections of the ovary one could see, under the suture, an elongated narrow cavity, filled with blood and outlined by a dark yellow wall. Close to this cavity and along the cortical there were small cysts similar to those described above (Fig. 6-21, No. 1982/62). *Omentum* - (Fig. 6-26) This looked normal, but one could disclose a richer vascular pattern. However, by palpation, it was possible to feel a very few minute hard granules (about 1 mm in size) surrounded by a radiary retraction of the omental tissue.

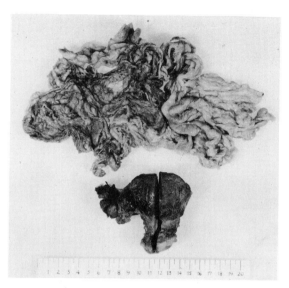

Fig. 6-26. No. 2476/62. - Total hysterectomy; the left adnexa had been previously removed. Normal sized uterus. Irregular serosal surface. In the upper part, the omentum: the nodules are not visible.

Microscopy Study: The uterine cervix and corpus did not show any particular changes. The endometrium was in the late proliferative phase. Every lesion described in the uterine and tubal serosa, on the ovarian surface and the omentum (Fig. 6-27) corresponded to malignant invasions, just as those described for the serosa of the left tube (No. 1982/62). In the sections of the right ovary an extensive reabsorption reaction was apparent around the suture threads. Nevertheless, the most striking images of these sections were (1) the presence of a recent corpus luteum, with hemorrhage, thus confirming the gross appearance, and (2) the luteinization and hyperplasia of the theca interna around the cysts, although less pronounced than in the wedge resected from this ovary (No. 1982/62, Fig. 6-24). The sections of the ampullar portion of the tubes showed marked hyperthrophy of the mucosa.

Comment: [2], [3], [5], [8-12], [15-26] The invasion of the uterine and tubal serosa, of the right ovary and the omentum just as previously described for the serosa of the left tube and left ovary, demonstrated the malignancy of the papillary outgrowths of the ovary. However, this malignancy was not hormonally active and cannot account for the virilizing syndrome. In the hilus of both ovaries no cells could be found which might explain the functional role played by these ovaries. It appears, therefore, that the only change observed in these ovaries was hyperthecosis.

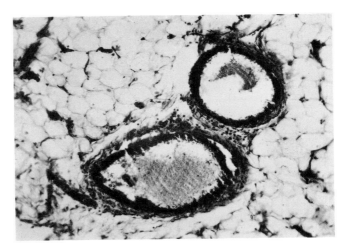

Fig. 6-27. No. 2477/62. H. Eos. 138x. - Omentum: malignant epithelium outlining small cavities, around which are small infiltrates.

CASE NO. IV: (#197.250)

M.J.V. - White female, age 23 years. She complained of menometrorrhagia during the last four months. Prior to this, in fact since the age of menarche, she menstruated normally. She also noticed a gradual onset of hirsutism, mainly in the face. There was no change in voice tone, but the breasts became smaller. Her physical examination was negative except for the presence of facial hirsutism (Fig. 6-28) and breast atrophy (Fig. 6-29). On pelvic examination she showed slight hypertrophy of the clitoris and a normal sized uterus. The right adnexa were enlarged: the ovary seemed to have the size of an orange.

Blood chemistry: N.P. nitrogen - 36 mg/100 ml.

Blood cytology: RBC. 4,020,000; WBC. - 8,200; hemoglobin 80 per cent.

Urine analysis: normal.

Hormone assays: 17 KS - 9.4 mg/24 hours; 17 KGS - 14.40 mg/24 hours; Estrone - 14.3 µg/24 hours; Estriol - 32.5 µg/24 hours. The stimulation test with 25 I.U. of corticotropin (ACTH), infused over an eight-hour period, on two successive days, resulted in a rise of the 17 KS to 18.6 mg/24 hours and of 17 KGS to 32.8 mg/24 hours. The patient was operated and the right adnexa, with an ovarian tumor, as well as a wedge of the left ovary, were removed. Two months following surgery the patient resumed normal monthly menses and noticed a sharp decrease in her hirsutism.

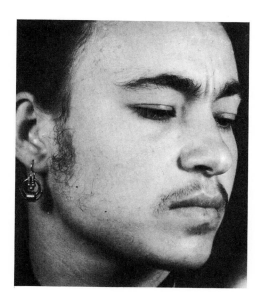

Fig. 6-28. M.J.V. - White female. Age 23. (#197.250).

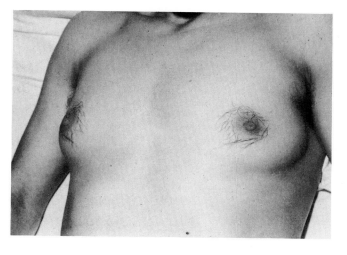

Fig. 6-29. M.J.V. - White female. Age 23. (#197.250).
Breast atrophy and hypertrichosis around the nipples.

PATHOLOGY REPORT

The right adnexa and a wedge resected from the left ovary were received for histopathologic study (Nos. 1.300/62 and 1.301/62, Feb. 6, 1962), with pre-operative diagnosis of : virilizing syndrome. Ovarian tumor?

Right Adnexa

Gross Appearance: Instead of the usual shape of the ovary the left ovary had a tumor the size of an orange, with a regular, smooth, round white-gray surface without adherences (Fig. 6-30). This tumor was very hard and did not show a rich vascularity. In its postero-superior and external face there was a cyst the size of a pigeon's egg,

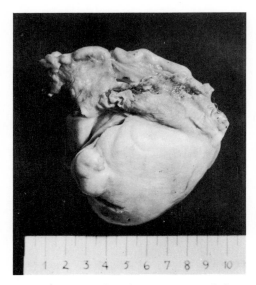

Fig. 6-30. No. 1300/62. - Right adnexa: tumor of the ovary, smooth round surface; to the upper left is the cyst. The tube is thin.

which had been previously opened and emptied; its inner surface was white and smooth, even where that surface touched the capsula of the tumor. A dense, brilliant tissue was seen in cross sections of the tumor. This was predominently yellow-white, in wide zones which rarely reached the capsula. To the periphery there was in smaller areas a dark brown tissue (Fig. 6-31). The capsula of this tumor which was not detachable, was thin, measuring in its thicker portion 2 mm. No cavities or cracks, necrotic or hemorrhagic zones were found in this tumor, which did not show any of the characteristics of the ovarian tissue. In the hilus and close to the capsula there were some dilated blood vessels. The macroscopic study showed that there was association of a solid tumor with a small ovarian cyst instead of a partly cystic tumor. The tube measured 8 cm and had a very narrow calliber; the infundibulum was normal. The tubal serosa was brilliant, smooth, and thin. The meso-salpinx was widened (Fig. 6-30), still preserving its usual thickness. No nodules or tumors could be felt by palpation. The tumor plus tube weighed 130 g.

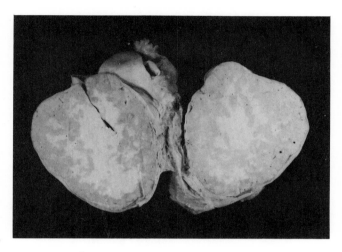

Fig. 6-31. No. 1300/62. – Ovarian tumor: cross section. Predominance of the yellow tissue (darker in this picture). More abundant clear fibrous tissue to the center with branches to the periphery. Thin capsula.

Microscopic Study: This is a rare tumor which had not been previously seen in this department. Serial sections were done and stained according to the following methods: Haemalumsn-Eosin, Van Gieson's, Masson's trichromic, and Tibor Papp's, besides the Sudan III in frozen sections. Extensive areas of fibrous tissue were frequently seen with collagen and hyalinization (Fig. 6-32). These were prolonged by bands and septs which divided into thinner branches, fibroblastic and more cellular, which sometimes gave rise to sarcoma-like images, if one considers as well the relationship between the vessels and the tissue. (Fig. 6-33). However, even in these sarcoma-like zones a careful examination could disclose other cellular types (Fig. 6-34). There were two main groups: one corresponded to typical lutein cells (Fig. 6-34 and 6-35); the other group was identifiable with Leydig cells, although it has not been possible to demonstrate Reinke's crystalloids. The above-mentioned cells were not seen limiting cavities or glandular tabules. However, a certain nodular or bundular pattern was apparent mainly in the trichromic (Fig. 6-37) and in the Tibor Papp stain (Fig. 6-39). The same pattern could also be demonstrated in the Sudan III stained sections which showed the lipid richness

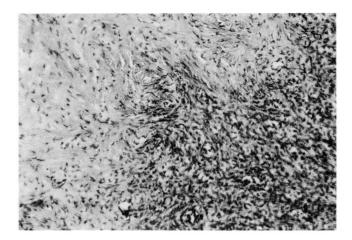

Fig. 6-32. No. 1300/62. H. Eos. 140x. - Change from the collagenous zone to the sarcomatoid tissue. Some "clear cells" can already be seen.

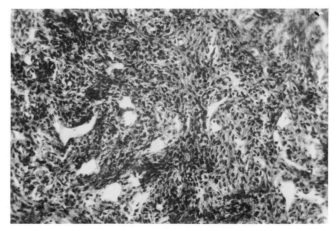

Fig. 6-33. No. 1300/62. H. Eos. 170x. - Sarcomatoid pattern. Many fibroblastic bundles forming the wall of the vessels and of some vascular spaces. "Clear cells" almost absent.

and abundance of lutein cells as well. (Fig. 6-36). In other fields (Fig. 6-35), which were almost exclusively formed by "epithelial" cells, close connections of the cells with sinusoidal capillaries were observed and could be said to be endocrinoid in type. There was a slight anisocariosis and hyperchromatism more evident in fibroblasts - sarcomatoid aspect - than in the "epithelial" cells. There were a few regular mitoses as well. These features did not support a diagnosis

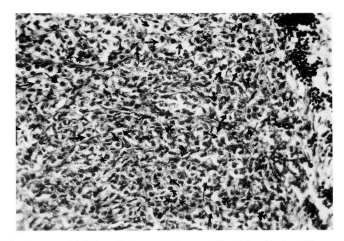

Fig. 6-34. No. 1300/62. H. Eos. 180x. - Fibroblastic bundles very rich in luteinized cells (arrows) and some Leydig cells (x).

of malignancy, in view of the perfect limits of the tumor which has no adherences to any surrounding structures. No ovarian tissue could be found in this tumor, which, as previously mentioned, did not display any tubular or glandular pattern. No teratoma or teratoid structures were seen. The cyst did not show any peculiarities; that is, its wall was not particularly thick and was fibrous and independent of the tumor capsula. The cyst was lined with a low, regular columnar epithelium. In the sections of the tube we could demonstrate a thin endosalpinx, low and slightly branched folds lined by a hypoplastic epithelium.

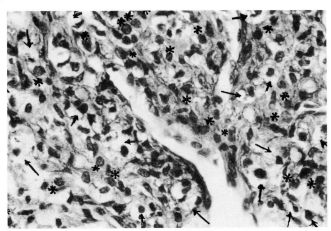

Fig. 6-35. No. 1300/62. H. Eos. 400x. - Many luteinized cells (arrows) and some Leydig cells (x). Sinusoid capillaries. "Endocrine type" blood supply. Scanty fibroblasts.

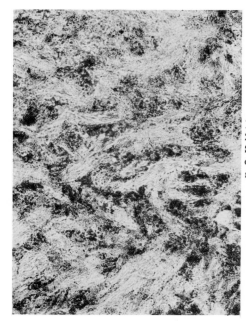

Fig. 6-36. No. 1300/62. Sudan III. 200x. - Many cells rich in lipoids (dark). Structure showing sometimes bundles, other times nodules. These images are similar in the thecoma.

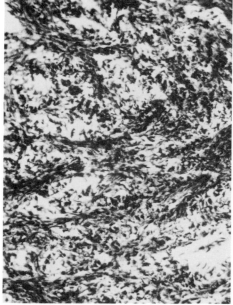

Fig. 6-37. No. 1300/62. Masson's trichromic stain. 200x. - Collagenous thick bundles. The epithelial-like cells form a strip-like structure.

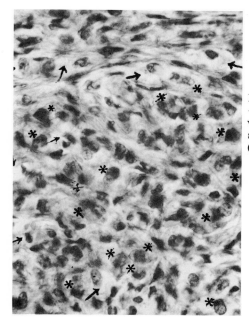

Fig. 6-38. No. 1300/62. H. Eos. 600x.
- Sarcomatoid immage. Fibroblasts
visible in the upper part. Anisocariosis,
scanty mitosis. A few luteinized cells
(arrows) and Leydig cells (x).

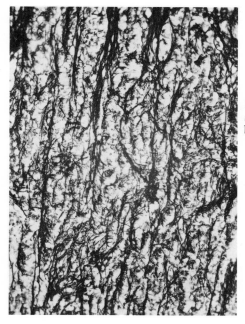

Fig. 6-39. No. 1300/62. Tibor Papp's
stain. 177x. - One can see, between
bundles of recticulin, rows of cells.

Left Ovary

(No. 1301/62) A fragment, the size of a small hazel, was received for examination (Fig. 6-40). The ovarian surface was smooth, grayish, and round; its opposite face was irregular and showed the wall of a cyst. In cross sections one could see slightly enlarged cysts separated by a clear, fibrous tissue, where no scars could be detected.
Microscopic Study: This showed follicular cysts with a thin granulosa cell layer, which was not present in some areas under a fibrous theca. In one of the cysts, which had been previously opened (Fig. 6-40), the granulosa cell layer was thin as compared to the theca, which showed hyperplasia with luteinization, hyperchromatism, and some mitoses. The tunica albuginea was fibrous. In some restricted areas of ovarian stroma there were a few primordial follicles. The remaining area of the sections showed fibrous tissue and some scars of corpora fibrosa, but no corpora lutea or its scars.

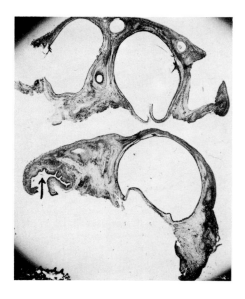

Fig. 6-40. No. 1301/62. H. Eos. 4x. - Left ovary: follicular cysts and diffuse fibrosis. In the lower right the albuginea (invisible and thin). In one cyst (arrow), hyperthecosis.

Comment: [2], [3], [5], [8-12], [15-26] The striking feature of this case was a solid, fibrous, yellow ovarian tumor which led us first to assume that we were dealing with a luteinized ovarian fibroma. On the other hand, the collagen richness, with areas of luteinization, as well as the distribution of the luteinized cells strongly, suggested the diagnosis of a thecoma. However, the thecoma has a feminizing biologic activity just like that of the granulosa cell tumor, both being included in the functioning mesenchimomas, according to Novak [19, 20]. This case was a virilizing syndrome. It should be said, nevertheless, that there have been reports in the literature of thecomas associated with virilism. The present case showed Leydig cells, as previously described, besides luteinized cells common to all "lipoid cell-virilizing tumors of the ovary." This finding led us to conclude that this was an arrhenoblastoma and not a thecoma, masculinovoblastoma, luteinoma, interstitioma, or adrenal cell rest tumor. The diagnosis could not be gynandroblastoma, since there was no association or mixture of morphologic elements common to granulosa cell tumors and thecomas with typical features of arrhenoblastoma.

Professor J.S. Horta from the University of Lisbon Medical School, who studied this material, agreed with the above diagnosis and suggested that it is incorrect to classify these cases as thecomas.

An arrhenoblastoma is a rare tumor, and establishing the diagnosis is always difficult since this tumor may display several morphological patterns. The clinical picture must be carefully considered. Norris [18] states that the diagnosis of an arrhenoblastoma cannot be based only on the pathology.

In the present case there is a good agreement between the clinical syndrome and the morphologic findings; the tumor is unilateral, solid, and bearing no adherences to other organs, which is characteristic of an arrhenoblastoma. The microscopic study shows that this is an undifferentiated arrhenoblastoma, a typical or sarcomatoid, falling in group III of Meyer's classifications; this is indeed the most frequently found pattern which is usually associated with virilism. Among the 114 cases of arrhenoblastoma reported by Hughesdon and Fraser and quoted by Hertig [9], thirteen (11.4 per cent) were undifferentiated (tubular adenoma of Pick), twenty-five (21.9 per cent) intermediate, and seventy-six (66.6 per cent) were undifferentiated or atypical. Although in this case no signs of malignancy could be found, Javert and Finn [12], among 122 cases collected from the literature and their own files, have found an incidence of malignancies of 22.9 per cent.

General references include the reports of the following workers: Barzilai [2], Blackman [3], Burket and Avel [5], Greenblatt, et al [8], Hertig and Gore [9], Horta [10], [10a], Iverson [11], Javert and Finn [12], Merivale and Forman [15], Meyer [16], Morris and Scully [17], Norris [18], Novak [19], [20], Novak and Gray [21], Novak and Novak [22], Plate [23], Stein and Leventhal [24], Sternberg and Gaskill [25], and Vernet [26].

DISCUSSION

Constitutional hirsutism is a definite entity that should be considered in every female, especially of Latin descent, with the following triad: (1) a long history of hirsutism with no sudden exacerbation of hair growth, (2) the absence of menstrual irregularities with a negative gynecological examination, and (3) the exclusion of ovarian, adrenal, and pituitary pathology.

Some of the difficulties encountered are those relating to the normal values for 17-ketosteroids observed in these patients. This, of course, does not exclude the actual presence of increased'levels of circulating androgens as clearly demonstrated by Dorfman (see Chapters 2, 3 and 4). The fact that testosterone is not a potent gonadotropin inhibitor (cf. Loraine in this book) may explain the frequent association of normally ovulatory menses with no other signs of virilization but hirsutism.

For the proper interpretation of hormone assays in hirsutism, the use of adrenal suppression tests is mandatory. Furthermore, ovarian stimulation tests with HCG (human chorionic gonadotropin) and employing dehydroepiandrosterone levels pre- and post-stimulation may help elucidate the diagnosis of ovarian factors responsible for hirsutism.

As for evaluation of adrenal factors, perirenal air insufflation does not always provide the desired information. We have adopted the clinical criterion of careful observation of patients with moderately elevated levels of 17-ketosteroids and 17-ketogenic steroids that can be suppressed with administered corticosteroids. The suppression should be such as to maintain normal or low levels of these steroids for at least three months. Unfortunately the prognosis of hirsutism is not very promising in the majority of cases. We have been able to decrease it, but not to suppress it entirely. Only in instances of virilizing tumors is the hirsutism completely reversible.

There is no pathognomonic pathological state of the polycystic ovary associated with hirsutism. There are probably many patients with polycystic ovaries resulting from adrenal dysfunction which can be adequately suppressed with exogenous corticoids. A wedge resection of these ovaries is not indicated. What really matters, however, is acceptance of the association of a common biochemical defect to the polymorphism of ovarian pathology associated with hirsutism, with a resulting high circulating level of androgens.

Finally, it can not be overemphasized that the clinician should always bear in mind the possibility of a malignancy as a cause of, or associated with, hirsutism.

The problem of hirsutism and virilizing syndromes is one which clearly confirms the need for endocrine-gynecologists, who may utilize the knowledge and technics of both specialties in a joint effort to diagnose and treat these patients.

Thanks are due to Doctors R. Iriarte Peixoto, M.D., Maria Luisa Martins Pereira, M.D., and Valentim de Carvalho, M.D., for referring some of these patients to us. We express our appreciation to Doctors Francisco Gentil Martins, M.D., Jose Cunha, M.D., and Ana Duarte, M.D., of the Department of Surgery.

REFERENCES

1. Appleby, J. I., and Norimberski, J. K. 1957. *J. Endocrinol.* 15: 310.
2. Barzilai, G. 1943. *Atlas of Ovarian Tumors.* Grune & Stratton, New York.
3. Blackmun, R. L. 1942. *Amer. J. Obstet. & Gynec.* 43: 1036.
4. Brown, J. B., Bulbrook, R. D., and Greenwood, F. C. 1957. *J. Endocrinol.* 16: 49.
5. Burket, J. A., and Abel, I. 1944. "Primary Masculinizing Tumors of the Ovary." *Surg. Gynec. Obstet.* 79: 651.
6. Fotherby, K. 1959. *Biochem. J.* 73: 339.
7. Fotherby, K., and Love, D. N. 1960. *J. Endocrinol.* 20: 157.
8. Greenblatt, R., et al. 1939. "Variations of Lipoid Content in Certain Ovarian Tumors." *Am. J. Obstet. & Gynec.* 37: 929.
9. Hertig, A. T., and Gore, H. 1961. *Tumors of the Female Sex Organs.* Part III, "Tumors of the Ovary and Fallopian Tube." Armed Forces Institute of Pathology, Washington, D. C.
10. Horta, J. S. 1945. "Tumores Feminizantes e Masculinizantes das Glandulas Sexuais." *Tokoginec. Pract.* 4: 161.
10a. Horta, J. S. 1947. "Tumores da Capsula Supra-Renal." *Liv. Luso-Espanhola,* ed. Lisboa.
11. Iverson, L. 1947. "Masculinizing Tumors of the Ovary." *Surg. Gynec. Obstet.* 84: 213.
12. Javert, C. T., and Finn, W. F. 1951. "Arrhenoblastoma. The Incidence of Malignancy and the Relationship to Pregnancy, to Sterility, and to Treatment." *Cancer* 4: 60.
13. Klopper, A., Michie, E., and Brown, J. B. 1955. *J. Endocrinol.* 12: 209.
14. Loraine, J. A., and Brown, J. B. 1959. *J. Endocrinol.* 18: 77.
15. Merivale, W. H. H., and Forman, L. 1951. "A Case of Masculin-ovoblastoma." *Brit. Med. J.* 1: 560.
16. Meyer, R. 1931. "The Pathology of Some Special Ovarian Tumors and Their Relation to Sex Characteristics." *Am. J. Obstet. & Gynec.* 22: 697.
17. Morris, J. M., and Scully, R. E. 1958. *Endocrine Pathology of the Ovary."* The C. V. Mosby Company, St. Louis.
18. Norris, E. H. 1938. "Arrhenoblastoma - A Malignant Ovarian Tumor Associated with Endocrinological Effects." *Am. J. Cancer* 50: 32.
19. Novak, E. 1948. "Functioning Tumors of the Ovary, with Special Reference to Pathology and Histogenesis." *J. Obstet. Gynaec. Brit. Emp.* 55: 725.
20. Novak, E. 1953. "Hormone-Producing Ovarian Tumors." *Obstet. & Gynec.* 1: 3.

21. Novak, E., and Gray, L.A. 1936. "Clinical and Pathological Differentiation of Certain Special Ovarian Tumors." *Am. J. Obstet. & Gynec.* **31**: 213.
22. Novak, E., and Novak, E.R. 1958. *Gynecologic and Obstetric Pathology*. W.B. Saunders & Co., Philadelphia & London.
23. Plate, W.P. 1958. "Pathologic Anatomy of the Stein-Leventhal Syndrome." *Fertil. & Steril.* **9**: 545.
24. Stein, J.F., and Leventhal, M.L. 1935. "Amenorrhea Associated with Bilateral Polycystic Ovaries." *Am. J. Obstet. & Gynec.* **29**: 181.
25. Sternberg, W.H., and Gaskill, C.J. 1950. "Theca-cell Tumors With a Report of Twelve New Cases and Observations on the Possible Etiologic Role of Ovarian Stromal Hyperplasia." *Am. J. Obstet. & Gynec.* **59**: 575.
26. Vernet, E.G., 1959. "Consideraciones sobre un caso de arrenoblastoma atipico." *Rev. Iber. Endocrinol.* **6**: 271.
27. Vestergaard, P. 1951. *Acta Endocrinol.* (Kbh.) **8**: 193.

VII

Robert B. Greenblatt, M.D., C.M.

THE STIMULATION OF OVULATION

For several decades the experimental induction of ovulation has been of considerable research interest. The ease with which ovulation may be stimulated in experimental animals has never been duplicated in humans. In the laboratory, gonadotropins of animal origin readily induce ovulation, but the results observed in animal experimentation could not be obtained clinically. The chemical induction of ovulation in both laboratory animals and humans has been attempted. When copper salts were injected intravenously in estrous rabbits, ovulation resulted, but this response failed in anestrous ones [16]. When a chemical agent, clomiphene, was administered to anovulatory women in a constant estrous state, ovulations were induced [31]. A promising new approach to the problem of ovulation has opened new avenues for the resolution of a most perplexing and stubborn process. Table 7-1 lists the methods now in vogue in management of ovulatory failure.

Table 7-1. Methods for Management of Ovulatory Failure

1. Correction of Psychophysical Disorders
2. Thyroid Medication
3. Pregnant Mares' Serum (PMSG) and/or Human Chorionic Gonadotrophin (HCG)
4. Radiation of the Pituitary and/or Ovaries
5. Estrogens and Progestogens (including Intravenous Estrogens)
6. Glucocorticoids
7. Wedge Resection of Polycystic Ovaries
8. Human Pituitary-FSH and HCG
9. Chemical Induction with Clomiphene (MRL-41)

CORRECTION OF PSYCHOPHYSICAL DISORDERS

Secondary amenorrhea, functional amenorrhea, and functional uterine bleeding are seen with frequency in individuals with emotional conflicts. Secondary amenorrhea in the young woman with anorexia nervosa or the compulsive neurotic whose anxiety for conception manifests itself in pseudocyesis are classic examples. For some, simple change of environment (the girl away from home at school, etc.) is sufficient to upset the hypothalamico-pituitary-ovarian axis. Fear, anxiety, or stress may result in hypothalamic amenorrhea. This was brought out in the study of the problem of amenorrhea in American WACS stationed in London during the Blitz of World War II. Amenorrhea is often a presenting symptom in women with disturbances in the nutritional state, whether it be malnutrition or obesity.

Functional uterine bleeding, just like amenorrhea, may be the result of psychophysical upsets. The psychosomatic aspects of functional uterine bleeding are well known. Correction of the psychophysical disorder is frequently rewarded by return of ovulatory menstrual cycles.

THYROID MEDICATION

Buxton and Southam, in their book *Human Infertility*, state that, "It is probably no exaggeration to say that the gynecologist in his treatment of menstrual abnormalities and infertility has administered more thyroid extract than the entire population of internists in their treatment of hypothyroidism in general" [9]. These authors consider the administration of thyroid extract to be a useless therapeutic procedure unless physical examination or one or more tests for thyroid activity suggest hypothyroidism. Many clinicians, adamant about not using steroids, readily administer thyroid medication, frequently beyond the level of tolerance, with the vague hope that there may be a generalized increase in metabolic activity which would regulate the menstrual dysfunction. Iatrogenic hypothyroidism is induced on cessation of thyroid medication. What seems to be forgotten is that because of this the patient now feels sluggish and tired. The physician, in restoring the patient to thyroid medication, ameliorates the new symptoms and compounds the error for which the therapy was intended [32].

Thyroid therapy is a most useful tool in the correction of menstrual abnormalities when there is an underlying disorder in thyroid function. Borderline hypothyroidism is frequently difficult to diagnose and the battery of tests now available is not always decisive. The basal metabolic rate is often misleading, the protein-bound iodine may be just above the lower limits of normal, the serum cholesterol may not be elevated, and the I^{131} uptake may be inconclusive. A one- or two-month therapeutic trial of thyroid medication in a dosage of 25 to 37.5 mcgm of 1-triiodothyronine or 60 to 90 mg of thyroid extract may be tried. If the results are disappointing, then cessation of further therapy should be advised. Larger doses of thyroid would only suppress

the endogenous thyroxin secretion and temporary iatrogenic hypothyroidism would set in when medication is discontinued.

GONADOTROPINS (OF ANIMAL ORIGIN) AND GONADOTROPIN-LIKE PREPARATIONS

Various types of gonadotropins have been commercially available.
Sheep pituitary extract, pregnant mares' serum, and chorionic gonadotropins derived from human pregnancy urine have been employed
singly, in combination, and in sequence.

The clinical use of human chorionic gonadotropin by American
workers has been uniformly unsuccessful in inducing ovulation [36].
However, the reports from Scandinavian countries on the successful
use of this hormone in cases of metropathia hemorrhagica cannot be
discounted. Bergman and Wahlen [2] pointed out that for HCG to produce desired results, the ovaries must contain fairly mature follicles.
When pregnant mares' serum gonadotropin (PMSG) become available,
Davis and Koff [12] presented their work which purported to show that
ovulation could be induced with this preparation. Their findings could
not be corroborated, but favorable results have been claimed for the
use of PMSG followed by HCG by Hamblen [37] and by Rydberg and
Pedersen-Bjergaard [55].

The concensus is that because of species specificity, gonadotropins of animal origin (sheep, calf, mare) are of little or no value in
the human. Chorionic gonadotropin derived from human pregnancy
urine (HCG) is of limited value alone but of considerable usefulness
when used in sequence to a course of human pituitary FSH.

IRRADIATION OF THE PITUITARY GLAND AND/OR OVARIES

Several decades ago, Dr. Ira Kaplan suggested the use of high-
voltage roentgen therapy in the treatment of amenorrhea and sterility
in women. Small-dosage irradiation of the pituitary gland and ovaries
has proved to be an effective form of therapy for the correction of
abnormalities of the menstrual rhythm, and this has been attested to
by Kaplan [45], [46], Israel [40], Rakoff [54], and many others. Rakoff,
however, has shown that the salutary results of irradiation to the pituitary and ovaries stem only from the response of the ovaries (Table
7-2). Although the benefits to be derived from irradiation therapy
have proved satisfactory in some hands, in other the results have been
poor and at times damaging. In some instances women with functional
amenorrhea have become totally amenorrheic. The fear of genetic
mutations in succeeding generations has limited the acceptance of such
a modality of treatment. Israel, once an enthusiastic proponent, is

now reluctant to employ irradiation therapy because he is convinced of
the hazards of ionizing radiation to future generations of mankind [52].

Table 7-2.   Low-Dosage Irradiation to Pituitary and Ovaries, and to
Ovaries Alone; Comparison of Results*

	Pituitary and ovaries		Ovaries alone	
	No.	Per cent	No.	Per cent
Number of patients	20		20	
Improved	12		11	
Estrogenic function	12	60	11	55
Corpus luteum function	9	45	8	40
Became pregnant	7	35	7	35
No change	7		6	
Made worse	1		3	

*From A. E. Rakoff, [54]

ESTROGENS AND/OR PROGESTOGENS

Zondek, at one time [64], suggested that small continuous estrogen
dosage might stimulate gonadotropin secretion from the pituitary. Large
doses have also been administered as a form of shock therapy to the
pituitary, i.e., to depress gonadotropin function in the hope of the occurrence of a sort of rebound phenomenon on cessation of medication.
Kupperman [48] has administered one to several intravenous Premarin
injections at monthly intervals, claiming that release of pituitary LH
thereby occurred.   Garcia and his associates [22] failed to corroborate
Kupperman's work and found that the occasional successes belonged to
the oligo-ovulators (Table 7-3).   Cyclic courses of estrogens and/or

Table 7-3.   Effect of Conjugated Estrogens (20 mg Intravenously) on
Ovulatory Failure*
(Mean age: 25.2; Median age: 27.5)

Diagnosis	No. of patients	Total no. of injections[†]	Total no. of ovulations
Anovulation	12	30	1
Oligo-ovulation	16	66	10[‡]

[†]At fourteen-day intervals
[‡]In six patients

*Reproduced from Garcia, et al., [22].

progestogens have been employed for many months in efforts to stimulate ovulation. Occasional favorable results have appeared after using various amounts and combinations. The best results were obtained in the management of women with metropathia hemorrhagica. After the arrest of bleeding with large doses of estrogens and/or progestogens, cyclic ovulatory menses frequently followed. In general, however, the relative infrequency of ovulations following gonadal steroids in both anovulators and oligo-ovulators, as well as the isolated pattern of incidence, suggests the lack of specificity of such agents.

CORTICOIDS

In 1950, Wilkins, et al. [63] showed that the administration of glucocorticoids suppressed abnormal adrenal steroid activity in females with congenital adrenal hyperplasia. Initiation of ovulatory menstruation occurred on satisfactory dosage. In 1953, Jones, Howard, and Langford [44] treated amenorrheic females with follicular phase defects and induced ovulatory menses in many. In the same year, Greenblatt [27] reported on the use of cortisone in hirsute amenorrheic females and found that ovulatory menses often followed such therapy. Since then, Perloff [53], Buxton [10], Jeffries [43], Gold [26], and many others have lent support to the theory of beneficial effects of corticoids in ovulatory failure, particularly when some degree of adrenal dysfunction was suspected. Recently, Lloyd [50], long skeptical as to the value of corticoids in such instances, has reversed his stand.

There are two possible explanations, which are not mutually exclusive, for the results obtained with corticoids in the treatment of menstrual abnormalities. The first of these explanations, which has not been emphasized in the literature, might be called the theory of balance of tropic pituitary hormones. In congenital adrenal hyperplasia, because of the inborn enzymatic disturbance, biosynthesis of cortisol and related compounds is considerably diminished or totally absent [1], [41], [42]. The lowering of the level of circulating cortisol will result in markedly increased ACTH secretion [60]. The supply of amino acids and peptides needed for the production of pituitary hormones seems to have different priorities upon this pool of materials. In malnutrition, gonadotropin production is the first to decrease. In severe anorexia nervosa, when all evidence of growth hormone, gonadotropic and thyrotropic activities are absent, corticotropic function still persists [30]. In congenital adrenal hyperplasia, with the outpouring of ACTH, the anterior pituitary reservoir of materials necessary for the manufacture of other hormones may become depleted, and so production of gonadotropins stops. Administration of glucocorticoids in adequate dosage arrests the manufacture of pituitary corticotropin, thereby releasing materials to the anterior pituitary reservoir and thus allowing for greater production and release of the other tropic hormones.

Thus gonadotropins will be released in greater quantity, permitting orderly ovarian function to take place [35].

The concept of increasing the release of pituitary gonadotropins by raising the blood levels of glucocorticoids finds support in the work of Sohval and Soffer [58], who have shown that the administration of ACTH or cortisone causes an immediate elevation of urinary gonadotropins. Furthermore, Davis and associates [13] administered ACTH to thirteen amenorrheic patients, and episodes of uterine bleeding were induced in nine of them. In some, bleeding occurred in spite of the rise in 17-ketosteroids and 17-hydroxycorticoids excretion. Moreover, Forsham and his collaborators [20] reported that three amenorrheic patients, who had not menstruated during the year, menstruated six to ten days after a single injection of 20 units of ACTH. Farnsworth [18] reported temporary re-establishment of regular menses in a 23-year-old amenorrheic girl with nephrosis following treatment with ACTH. These observations seem to indicate that both ACTH and cortisone administration may depress pituitary corticotropin activity and thus permit a better balance in the production and secretion of other pituitary hormones, and that in certain cases the effectiveness of cortisone may not be dependent solely upon the reduced androgen and/or estrogen secretion by the adrenals.

In Wilkins' hypothesis, which is based on frank cases of congenital adrenal hyperplasia [3], [4], [7], [15], the increased secretion of 17-ketosteroids and pregnanetriol is related to an abnormality in the biosynthesis of adrenal steroids. The cause of this is lack of specific enzymes with consequent alteration in normal metabolic pathways of cortisol synthesis. Cortisol production is considerably reduced or absent. The removal of the regulating action of this steroid on the pituitary leads to excessive output of corticotropin. This in turn stimulates the abnormally functioning adrenal cortex to produce excessive amounts of steroids other than cortisol. The excess secretion of androgen and/or estrogen by the adrenal cortex is thought to inhibit gonadotropin production and thereby to induce amenorrhea.

WEDGE RESECTION OF POLYCYSTIC OVARIES (STEIN-LEVENTHAL SYNDROME)

In 1935, Stein and Leventhal [59] reported on the polycystic ovary syndrome and the correction of the accompanying menstrual disorder by wedge resection of the ovaries. If certain criteria are met in the selection of patients, e. g., the demonstration of bilaterally enlarged ovaries in hirsute anovulatory females with menstrual disorders, then adequate wedge resection of the ovaries is usually followed by satisfactory regulation of the menstrual cycle. Many clinicians have attested to the benefits of this procedure.

The Stein-Leventhal syndrome is a form of hyperovarianism which is most likely caused by increased responsiveness of the ovaries to endogenous gonadotropins. The reduction of ovarian mass, whether by ignipuncture, wedge resection, removal of one ovary, or irradiation, would make more LH available per unit of ovarian mass, and thus permit ovulation to occur [28].

Although the clinical picture is similar in most women diagnosed as having Stein-Leventhal syndrome, there are, nevertheless, many variants of this entity. The response of patients to wedge resection of the ovary suggests that the abnormality in the ovaries may be the cause of the syndrome. This belief is supported by the fact that there is a marked decrease in the levels of urinary androsterone and etiocholanolone following wedge resection [38]. On the other hand, the findings of elevated levels of urinary steroids such as pregn-5-ene-3β, 17α, 20α-triol, heretofore considered to be of adrenal origin [11], [21] seemed to implicate abnormal function of the adrenals as the possible cause of the syndrome.

The Stein-Leventhal syndrome is primarily an ovarian disorder. The protagonists for the adrenal origin of this disturbance find it difficult to explain why good results should be obtained by wedge resection. Aside from the excellent results accomplished in many by reduction of ovarian mass through surgery, certain patients with this syndrome also respond to corticoid administration or to agents which influence or modify pituitary-ovarian relationships. Among the latter are HP-FSH followed by HCG and nonsteroidal agents such as clomiphene.

HUMAN PITUITARY FSH AND HCG

The first investigator to use HP-FSH successfully was Gemzell. He induced ovulation by administering a partially purified human pituitary FSH followed by HCG in 29 of 40 amenorrheic women [23], [25]. The work was confirmed by Buxton and Herrmann [8], who in like manner induced ovulation in six of seven amenorrheic women and in another by HCG alone. Although Greenblatt and Mahesh [33] were able to induce secretory endometria and numerous corpora lutea in the ovaries of amenorrheic women by HP-FSH followed by HCG, they were unable to stimulate ovulation with HP-FSH alone. In several cases, HCG was administered at the same time as HP-FSH (as a measure of expediency). Such a regimen proved nonbeneficial, and it was felt that sequential therapy would be more logical and preferable. Much has yet to be learned as to proper choice of patient, correct dosage, and the timing of administration of human gonadotropins in order to reproduce the cyclic changes which normally take place. However, Gemzell [24] claims that he has finally succeeded in a high percentage of his cases by modifying his previously employed dosage schedule.

CHEMICAL INDUCTION OF OVULATION

Various nonsteroid substances have been reported to induce ovulation in animals. Fevold, et al. [19] noted that injection of yeast extracts and copper salts caused ovulation in immature rabbits. Bradbury [5] showed that following induction of ovulation by copper salt the hypophyseal gonadotropin was depleted. Emmens [17] found that various salts of cadmium would produce ovulation in laboratory animals.

Successful induction of ovulation in six of 18 anovulatory women was reported by Tyler, et al. [62] following the administration of a nonsteroid antiestrogenic agent related to chlorotrianisene (TACE) and known as MER-25. The authors felt that in these patients the levels of estrogens were too constant to allow for cyclic pituitary activity. Incidentally, three of the six patients conceived [61]. The observations with MER-25 were confirmed by Kistner and Smith [47]. They reported four cases with Stein-Leventhal syndrome who were treated with this agent for varying periods. All four of them ovulated and two became pregnant. Because of its toxicity, MER-25 is no longer available for clinical trial. However, a new synthetic compound, clomiphene, was found to have the unexpected potential of modifying pituitary activity by the induction of ovulatory-type menstruation in 70 to 75 per cent of the amenorrheic women who were subjected to therapeutic trials [29], [31], [34] (Table 7-4).

Table 7-4. Clomiphene for Induction of Ovulation

	Patients treated		Ovulated				Failure				Side effects		Conception
			With menses		Without menses		No menses		Anovulatory menses		Cystic ovary	Hot flshs	
	#pts	#cyc	#pts	#cyc	#pts	#cyc	#pts	#cyc	#pts	#cyc			
Functional amenorrhea	56	283	48	198	1	1	6	21	1	2	8	5	15
Secondary amenorrhea	48	311	27	117	4	12	13	52	4	12	8	5	5
Primary amenorrhea	11	70	3	19	-	-	7	23	1	12	5	2	-
Stein-Leventhal syndrome	35	134	32	117	-	-	3	4	-	-	10	4	6
Functional uterine bleeding	26	141	22	107	1	1	1	1	2	5	4	1	2
Miscellaneous	3	17	-	-	1	4	1	2	1	2	-	-	-
Total	179	956	132	558	7	18	31	103	9	33	35	17	28

pts = patients   cyc = cycles

Clomiphene is also structurally related to chlorotrianisene (Fig. 7-1). In the rat, Holtkamp, et al. [39], and Segal and Nelson [56] found that it possessed antifecundity properties. In the human, clomiphene has a wide spectrum of activity. It is thought to be antiestrogenic because regressive changes were induced in the vaginal mucosa of children with precocious puberty. It may be assumed to have either antiestrogenic activity or the ability to cause autonomic nervous system imbalance because hot flashes were induced in about 10 per cent of the patients. It has luteotropic properties, for when administered

CHLOROTRIANISENE (TACE)

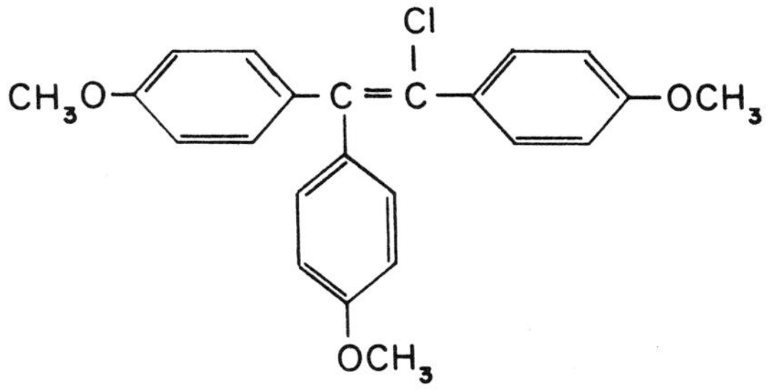

Chlorotris (p - methoxyphenyl) ethylene

CLOMIPHENE (MRL - 41)

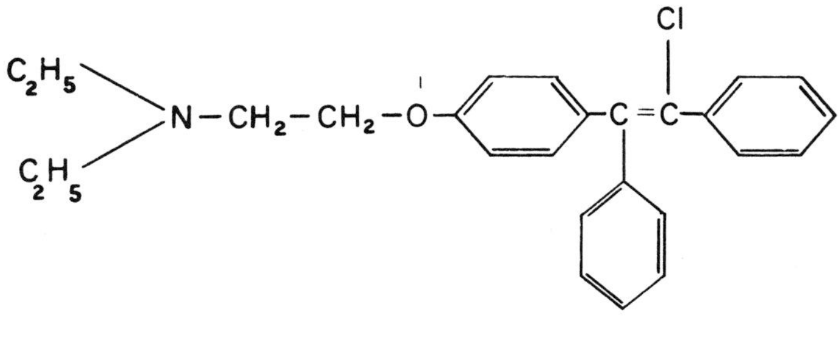

1 - [p (β-diethylaminoethoxy) phenyl] - 1, 2 -diphenyl-
2-chloroethylene

Fig. 7-1. Note similarities in structure between TACE and clomiphene

to women with a short ovulatory phase, the basal body temperature (BBT) was sustained in the luteal phase for 21 days (Figs. 7-2a and 7-2b). It has LH-like activity, for in nonhirsute as well as hirsute women with functional or secondary amenorrhea, clomiphene was capable of inducing ovulatory-type menses in 70 to 75 per cent of the

P.S.B.– w.f.– age 26– Inadequate Luteal Phase

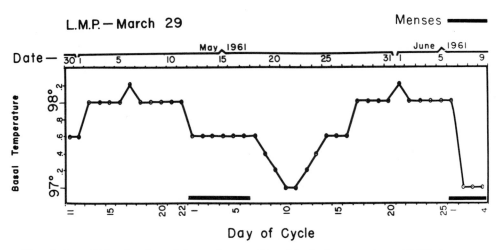

Fig. 7-2a.   Note short ovulatory phase.   Basal body temperature (BBT) is elevated for about ten days in a 26-year-old female.   (Reproduced from [29].)

P.S.B.– w.f.– age 26— Sustained Luteal Phase

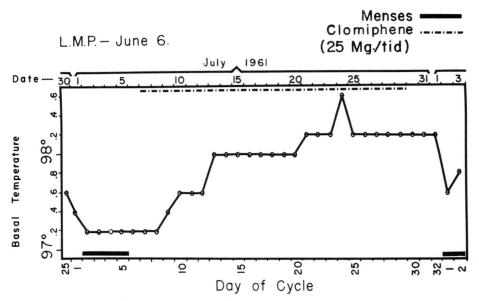

Fig. 7-2b.   Note sustained elevation of BBT in the luteal phase while the patient was on clomiphene therapy.

anovulatory women, as judged by the thermogenic shift in basal temperature and secretory changes in the endometrium (Fig. 7-3).

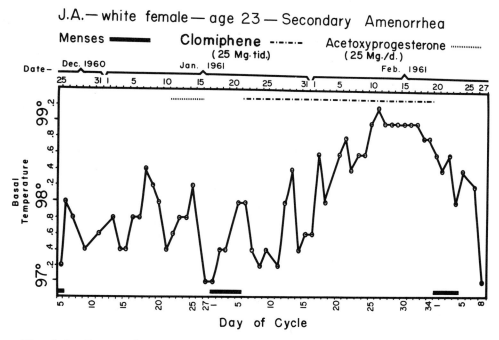

Fig. 7-3. Note ovulatory rise in BBT following a course of clomiphene in a 23-year-old female with secondary amenorrhea in whom withdrawal uterine bleeding was induced at monthly intervals with a progestin.

Thus far, 28 pregnancies in this series may be attributed to the ovulatory stimulating effects of the drug (Fig. 7-4). It is not an estrogen, for it did not cause maturation of the atrophic vaginal mucosa of menopausal women. It is not a progestin, for it did not induce bleeding after a five-day course of therapy in estrogen-primed amenorrheics. It is not an androgen, for no masculinizing effects were noted on prolonged therapy. It is not a glucocorticoid, for it did not suppress adrenal function.

How does clomiphene work? Where is the site of action of this drug? How does one account for its biologic activities? These are important questions which still require an answer. For the present, it is apparent that this agent is a pituitary modifier, having at least two actions. Clomiphene is capable of inducing ovulatory-like menses and of sustaining the corpus luteum for periods longer than the usual 14-day luteal phase.

The proper sequence and admixture of FSH and LH are necessary for ovulation. The maintenance of the corpus luteum is attributed to the luteotropic hormone. A sustained effect may be obtained by the administration of large doses of HCG during the luteal phase [6]. It may be assumed that clomiphene either alters the synthesis of pituitary gonadotropins or plays a significant part in their release. That its action may be mediated through the central nervous system (hypothalamic or autonomic) may be surmised by the frequent occurrence of hot flashes during medication.

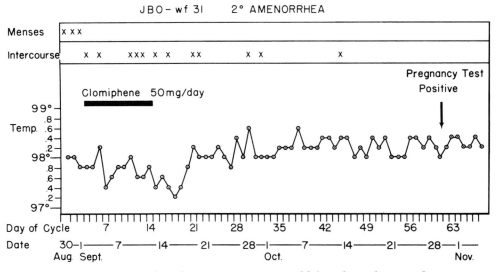

Fig. 7-4. Induction of ovulation in a 31-year-old female with secondary amenorrhea of long duration. Short courses of clomiphene were followed by a secondary thermogenic rise in BBT. Conception followed and she was delivered of a normal male infant.

It appears that clomiphene exerts antiestrogenic effects in human beings and that the suppression of the estrogenic end of the pituitary-ovarian system of feedback may be the means of exciting enough pituitary activity to bring on ovulation. That pituitary release may be achieved through interference with the enzyme system involved in the reversible estradiol to estrone reaction has been suggested by Olive Smith [57]. It is also possible that the pituitary releasing effect of clomiphene may be directly mediated through the hypothalamus. An analogy may be drawn from the occurrence of either ovulation or pseudopregnancy in rabbits and cats following electrical stimulation of the hypothalamus or of the hypophyseal stalk [14]. Furthermore, the induction of ovulation with clomiphene in two patients with Chiari-Frommel syndrome (persistent lactation, amenorrhea, and hypoestrogenism as manifested by a castrate type of vaginal cytology and an atrophic endometrium) suggests a direct action on the hypothalamico-pituitary axis [34].

The ovarian stimulating effect of clomiphene is not unlike that which follows a course of HP-FSH or sequential HP-FSH-HCG administration. The cystic ovaries frequently produced by clomiphene (Figs. 7-5a and 7-5b) compare in size and appearance both grossly and histologically with those often produced by human gonadotropins (Figs. 7-6a and 7-6b) [51].

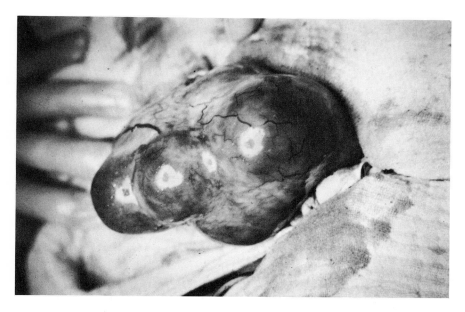

Fig. 7-5a. Enlarged cystic ovaries were found at laparotomy in a patient with Stein-Leventhal syndrome following a course of HP-FSH and HCG.

In spite of the high incidence of 25 per cent proved and presumed cyst formation of one or both ovaries, it is the considered opinion of the author that clomiphene is exceedingly worthwhile. Though this complication may be cause for concern, cessation of therapy and lapse of time (several weeks) will resolve the problem. This untoward effect must not overshadow the remarkable results obtained with this pituitary-modifying agent. In order to minimize this complication, the suggestion is put forward that clomiphene be administered in the dosage range of 25 to 50 mg per day (75 to 100 mg per day in resistant cases) and administered until ovulation occurs or for 30 to 90 days. If a response is not obtained, then further trial is usually worthless. Where a pattern of ovulation is established, then the dosage range may be reduced to courses of five to ten days in each cycle. The results so far obtained with clomiphene seem to give promise of a major advance in the treatment of ovulatory disorders.

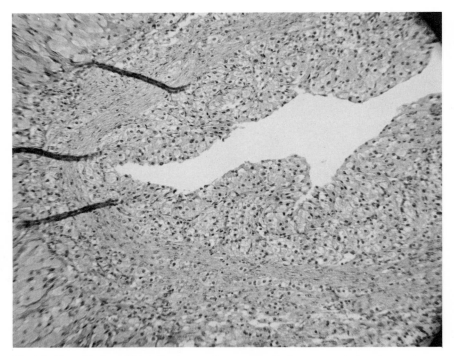

Fig. 7-5b. Study of histologic sections revealed corpora lutea in various stages of development. Note luteinized granulosa and theca cells.

SUMMARY AND CONCLUSIONS

The induction of ovulation is one of the areas of human reproduction which has met with little and varied success. Stimulating doses of irradiation to the pituitary and/or ovaries, in some hands, has been found useful, but advocates of this method are few because of reservations concerning gene mutations that may result from such manipulations. Wedge resection of the ovaries has proved a valuable procedure in the management of the Stein-Leventhal syndrome through the reduction of ovarian mass. The administration of glucocorticoids has been shown to have some merit in women with follicular phase defects and in certain amenorrheic females with hirsutism. The ideal hormones for the induction of ovulation would be human pituitary follicle-stimulating hormone (HP-FSH) followed by a course of human luteinizing

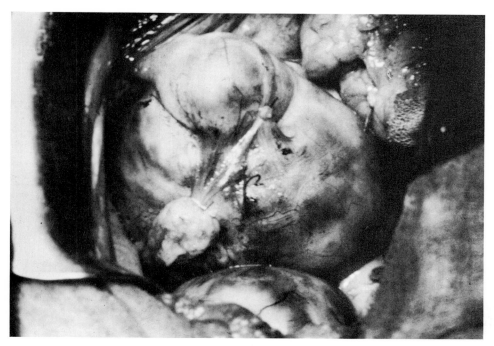

Fig. 7-6a.   Large cystic ovaries were found at laparotomy in patient with Chiari-Frommel syndrome following an extensive and prolonged course of clomiphene.

hormone (LH).   Actually, HP-FSH and human chorionic gonadotrophin (HCG) have been satisfactorily employed experimentally, but the scarcity of human FSH precludes its clinical adoption.

Occasionally, cyclic estrogens and/or progestogens have been used in functional amenorrhea to restore pituitary-ovarian balance with isolated instances of success.   Striking results are frequently obtained with thyroid medication in the subclinical hypothyroid patient with ovulatory failure.   The correction of psychophysical disorders has proved rewarding.   But one of the most important developments in reproductive physiology was the introduction for experimental purposes of a new synthetic chemical agent, clomiphene (MRL-41), which has the remarkable potential of modifying pituitary activity by the induction of ovulation in a high percentage of anovulatory women.

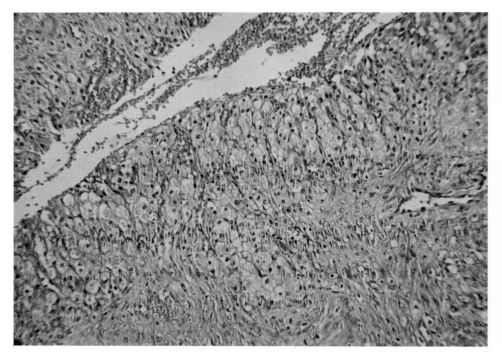

Fig. 7-6b.   Histologic sections revealed corpora lutea in various stages of development.   Note similarity of response to that obtained in Figure 7-5b.

REFERENCES

1. Barter, F.C., Albright, F., Forbes, A.P., Leaf, A., Dempsey, E., and Carroll, E. 1951. *J. Clin. Invest.* **30**: 237.
2. Bergman, P., and Wahlen, T. 1952. *Acta Endocrinol.* **9**: 69.
3. Bongiovanni, A.M. 1953. *Bull. Johns Hopkins Hosp.* **92**: 244.
4. Bongiovanni, A.M., Eberlein, W.R., and Cara, J. 1954. *J. Clin. Endocrinol.* **14**: 409.
5. Bradbury, J.T. 1944. *Am. J. Physiol.* **142**: 487.
6. Brown, W.E., and Bradbury, J.T. 1947. *Am. J. Obstet. & Gynec.* **53**: 749.
7. Butler, G.C., and Marrian, G.F. 1937. *J. Biol. Chem.* **119**: 565.
8. Buxton, C.L., and Herrmann, W. 1961. *Am. J. Obstet. & Gynec.* **81**: 584.
9. Buxton, C.L., and Southam, A.L. 1958. *Human Infertility,* Paul B. Hoeber, Inc., New York.

10. Buxton, C. L., and Vande Wiele, R. L. 1954. *New Eng. J. Med.* 251: 293.
11. Cox, R. I., and Shearman, R. P. 1961. *J. Clin. Endocrinol. & Metab.* 21: 586.
12. Davis, M. E., and Koff, A. K. 1938. *Am. J. Obstet. & Gynec.* 36: 183.
13. Davis, M. E., Test, C. E., Navori, C. A., Hayse, B., Pottenger, R. E. and Dunkle, F. 1952. *J. Clin. Endocrinol.* 12: 696.
14. Dey, F. L. 1943. *Endocrinology* 33: 75.
15. Dorfman, R. I. 1955. *Ciba Found. Colloq. on Endocrinol.* 8: 112.
16. Dury, A., and Bradbury, J. T. 1943. *Am. J. Physiol.* 139: 135.
17. Emmens, G. W. 1940. *J. Endocrinol.* 2: 63.
18. Farnsworth, E. B. 1950. *First Clinical ACTH Conference*, J. R. Mote, ed., Blakiston Co., Philadelphia, 297.
19. Fevold, H. L., et al. 1936. *Am. J. Physiol.* 117: 68.
20. Forsham, P. H., Thorn, G. W., Prunty, F. T. G., and Hills, A. G. 1948. *J. Clin. Endocrinol.* 8: 15.
21. Gallagher, T. F., Kappas, A., Hellman, L., Lipsett, M. B., Pearson, O. H., and West, C. D. 1958. *J. Clin. Invest.* 37: 794.
22. Garcia, C. R., Harrigan, J. T., Mulligan, W. J., and Rock, J. 1960. *Fertil. & Steril.* 11: 303.
23. Gemzell, C. A. 1960. *Ciba Found. Colloq. on Endocrinol.* 13: 191.
24. Gemzell, C. A. 1962. Personal communication.
25. Gemzell, C. A., Diczfalusy, E., and Tillinger, G. 1958. *J. Clin. Endocrinol. & Metab.* 18: 1333.
26. Gold, J. J. 1958. *Am. J. Obstet. & Gynec.* 75: 1034.
27. Greenblatt, R. B. 1953. *Am. J. Obstet. & Gynec.* 66: 700.
28. Greenblatt, R. B. 1961. *Maryland State M. J.* 10: 1.
29. Greenblatt, R. B. 1961. *Fertil. & Steril.* 12: 402.
30. Greenblatt, R. B., Barfield, W. E., and Clark, S. L. 1951. *J. M. A. Ga.* 40: 299.
31. Greenblatt, R. B., Barfield, W. E., Jungck, E. C., and Ray, A. W. 1961. *J. A. M. A.* 178: 101.
32. Greenblatt, R. B., Clark, S. L., and Lord, J. R. 1960. *Clin. Obstet. & Gynec.* (Dec.), 1006, Paul B. Hoeber, Inc. New York.
33. Greenblatt, R. B., and Mahesh, V. B. 1961. Abstr. 43rd Ann. Meeting, Endocrine Soc.
34. Greenblatt, R. B., Mahesh, V. B., and Roy, S. 1962, *Am. J. Obstet. & Gynec.* 84: 900.
35. Greenblatt, R. B., Martinez-Manautou, J., Clark, S. L., and Rosenberg, A. P. 1958. Metabolism 7: 25.
36. Greenblatt, R. B., and Pund, E. R. 1941. *South. Med. J.* 34: 730.
37. Hamblen, E. C., and Davis, C. D. 1945. *Am. J. Obstet. & Gynec.* 50: 137.
38. Herrmann, W., Buckner, F., and Morris, J. M. 1960. *Fertil. & Steril.* 11: 74.

39. Holtkamp, D., Davis, R. H., and Rhoada, J. E. 1961. *Fed. Proc.* 20: 419.
40. Israel, S. L. 1952. *Am. J. Obstet. & Gynec.* 64: 971.
41. Jailer, J. W. 1953. *Bull. N. Y. Acad. Med.* 29: 377.
42. Jailer, J. W. 1955. *Int. Med.* 7: 1125.
43. Jeffries, W. M. 1962. *J. Clin. Endocrinol. & Metab.* 22: 255.
44. Jones, G. E. S., Howard, J. E., and Langford, H. 1953. *Fertil. & Steril.* 1: 49.
45. Kaplan, I. I. 1948. *Am. J. Roentg.* 59: 370.
46. Kaplan, I. I. 1958. *Am. J. Obstet. & Gynec.* 76: 447.
47. Kistner, R. W., and Smith, O. W. 1961. *Fertil. & Steril.* 12: 121.
48. Kupperman, H. S., et al. 1958. *Fertil. & Steril.* 9: 26.
49. Kurzrok, R., Wilson, L., and Cassidy, M. A. 1935. *Am. J. Obstet. & Gynec.* 29: 771.
50. Lloyd, C. 1962. Personal communication.
51. Mahesh, V. B., and Greenblatt, R. B. 1961. *Nature* 191: 888.
52. Mazer, C., and Israel, S. L. 1959. *Menstrual Disorders and Sterility*, 4th ed., Paul B. Hoeber, Inc., New York.
53. Perloff, W. H., Channick, B. J., Hadd, H. E., and Nodine, J. H. 1958. *Fertil. & Steril.* 9: 247.
54. Rakoff, A. E. 1953. *Fertil. & Steril.* 4: 263.
55. Rydberg, E., and Pedersen-Bjergaard, K. 1943. *J. A. M. A.* 121: 1117.
56. Segal, S. J., and Nelson, W. O. 1961. *Anat. Rec.* 139: 273.
57. Smith, O. 1962. *J. A. M. A.* (Letter to Editor) 179: 99.
58. Sohval, A. R., and Soffer, L. J. 1951. *J. Clin. Endocrinol.* 11: 677.
59. Stein, I. F., and Leventhal, M. L. 1935. *Am. J. Obstet. & Gynec.* 29: 181.
60. Sydnor, K. L., Kelley, V. C., Raile, R. B., Ely, R. S., and Sayers, G. 1953. *Proc. Soc. Exper. Biol. Med.* 82: 695.
61. Tyler, E. T. Personal communication.
62. Tyler, E. T., Olson, H. J., and Gotlib, M. H. 1960. *Internat. J. Fertil.* 5: 429.
63. Wilkins, L., Lewis, R. A., Klein, K., and Rosemberg, E. 1950. *Bull. Johns Hopkins Hosp.* 86: 249.
64. Zondek, B., Personal communication.

VIII

Robert B. Greenblatt, M.D., C.M.
THE INHIBITION OF OVULATION

The inhibition of ovulation as a therapeutic tool, first suggested by Wilson, was introduced into clinical practice by Sturgis and Albright in 1940 [26]. In the management of dysmenorrhea, the administration of 1.66 mg of estradiol benzoate intramuscularly on days 7, 10, and 13 of the cycle was followed by a painless, anovulatory bleeding period at about the anticipated time, i.e., the 28th day. However, on repetition of the estrogen therapy in the succeeding cycle, the dysmenorrhea recurred because ovulation had intervened before the second course of hormonal therapy could prove effective. In 1954 the author reported on the continuous administration of estrogens to circumvent "ovulation-escape" that occurred when estrogens were given either in short courses parenterally early in the cycle or orally from day 5 to day 25 of the cycle. Inhibition of ovulation was successfully induced for periods of 12 months. Small doses of a progestational agent were superimposed for two to three days at monthly intervals to induce withdrawal bleeding periods and thus prevent or minimize the chances of breakthrough bleeding. This regimen proved particularly successful in the management of the difficult-to-control membranous dysmenorrhea [14].

In 1956 Rock, Garcia, and Pincus [24] reported before the Laurentian Hormone Conference the successful inhibition of ovulation for months on end by the cyclic use of the 19-norsteroids from day 5 to day 25. The implication was that a new measure for the control of conception was in the offering. In 1957 a preliminary report by Rice-Wray [22] appeared which gave the results of a study initiated by the Family Planning Association of Puerto Rico on the efficacy and safety of norethynodrel with ethinyl estradiol 3 methyl ether for ovulation control. Since then, many studies have corroborated the utility of antiovulatory drugs in prevention of conception [3], [6], [7], [19], [20], [21], [23], [25], [27], [28].

Limiting the size of the family has been an age-old dream practiced in one form or another by diverse peoples in different civilizations. American Indian women believed, and still do, that the ingestion of certain herbs such as lithospermum ruderole will prevent conception. Since the advent of the 19-norsteroids much progress has been made in this field of endeavor.

The ideal agent for the prevention or delay of the due process of ovulation has been a goal sought by modern-day students of reproductive physiology. It should be stressed, however, that antiovulatory drugs also have been employed to great advantage in the management of severe mittelschmerz, essential dysmenorrhea, severe premenstrual tension, membranous dysmenorrhea, endometriosis, and hypermenorrhea, and to rest the pituitary-ovarian axis in the hope of overcoming sterility. Nevertheless, the greatest potential for these agents lies in the control of conception [8].

ANTIOVULATORY AGENTS

The antiovulatory drugs listed below have been employed in clinical studies by Greenblatt's group at the Medical College of Georgia [2], [4], [10], [11], [12], [13], [15]. Note that all but norethindrone were supplemented with an estrogen. EE3ME refers to ethinyl estradiol 3 methyl ether, and EE to ethinyl estradiol.

Enovid®	Norethynodrel with EE3ME
Norlutin®	Norethindrone
Dimethisterone®	6α-methyl-17 (1-propynyl) testosterone with EE
Provera®	6α-methyl-17α-acetoxyprogesterone with EE
Chlormadinone®	6-chloro Δ^6-17α-acetoxyprogesterone with EE3ME
Duphaston®	6-dehydro-retroprogesterone with EE
Norlutate®	Norethindrone acetate with EE
Gestagen®	Allylestrenol with stilbestrol

The chemical structure of these agents permits them to be grouped into three classes, and some of them have been arranged to show their visual relationships to one another.

1. Estrane derivatives with progestational activity such as norethynodrel, norethindrone, norethindrone acetate and allylestrenol. All of these may be said to be 19-norsteroids in that there is absence of a 19-methyl group. Their chemical configuration bears a resemblance to estradiol, a pure estrogen (Fig. 8-1).

2. Androstane derivatives with progestational activity such as ethisterone and dimethisterone. Compare structure to testosterone and dimethisterone. Compare structure to testosterone and methyltestosterone, potent androgenic substances. Note the close relationship of norethindrone, a potent progestational agent in Group 1, to ethisterone (Fig. 8-2).

3. Pregnane derivatives with progestational activity such as Provera®, chlormadinone, and Duphaston®. All of these are C 21 compounds comparable to progesterone (Fig. 8-3).

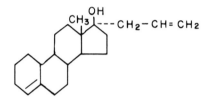

Estradiol

Norethynodrel

Norethindrone

Allylestrenol

Fig. 8-1. Estrane derivatives with progestational
activity. Note structural relationship to estradiol.

It should be emphasized that the progestational agents are administered in combination with an estrogen in order to have antiovulatory
propensities. Norlutin®, as it is now constituted, contains an estrogen
contaminant, hence its effectiveness.

INDICATIONS

Several conditions common in gynecologic practice require knowl-
edgeable and working acquaintance with antiovulatory agents for their
successful management. Some of these conditions will be discussed
under individual headings.

Membranous Dysmenorrhea

The term "membranous dysmenorrhea" refers to the painful passage of an endometrial cast of the uterus. This usually occurs sometime during the first few days of menstruation. The endometrial cast

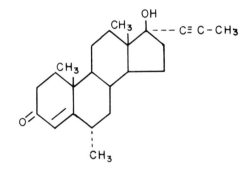

Testosterone

Methyltestosterone

Ethisterone

Dimethisterone

Fig. 8-2. Androstane derivatives with progestational activity. Note structural relationship to testosterone and methyl testosterone.

oftentimes is referred to as a decidual cast because of the pronounced decidual reaction noted on histologic study. Many of the cases go unrecognized because the cast is passed in fragments and the patient merely complains of severe dysmenorrhea in association with passage of large clots. If the index of suspicion is great enough, the physician may give the patient a bottle containing 10 per cent formalin in which to save these so-called clots. The diagnosis may thus be made with greater frequency. Since the introduction of potent 19-norsteroids the occurrence of decidual casts has become common. Progesterone has this same property, and large doses administered for 15 to 30 days have been followed by the passage of a decidual cast.

The successful management of patients with membranous dysmenorrhea by the continuous suppression of ovulation was established, as previously mentioned, by the author in 1954 [14]. Ovulation was suppressed or delayed through the administration of oral conjugated

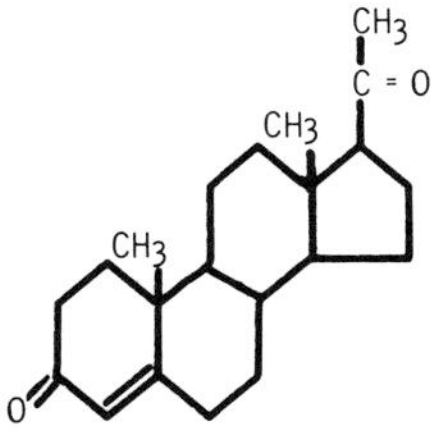

Progesterone

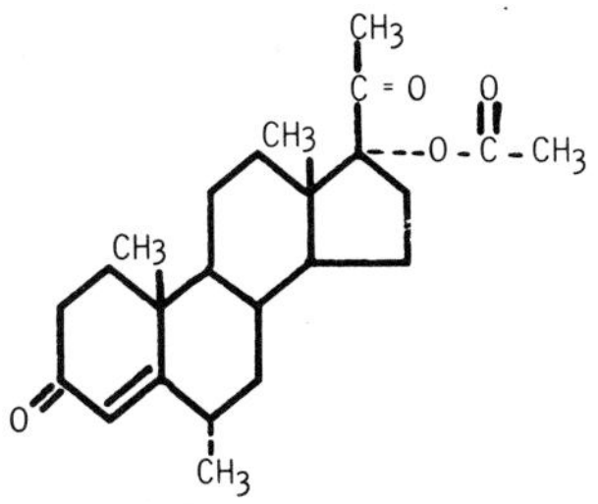

6 – Methyl 17 – acetoxy progesterone
(Provera)

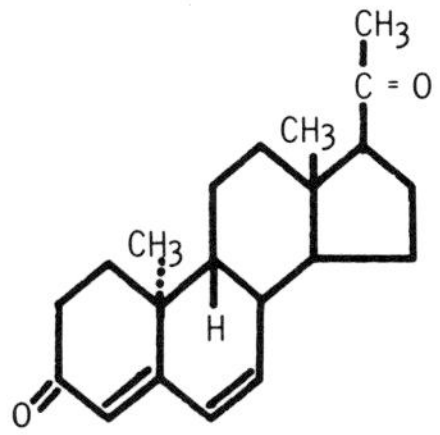

6 - dehydro - retro - progesterone
(Duphaston)

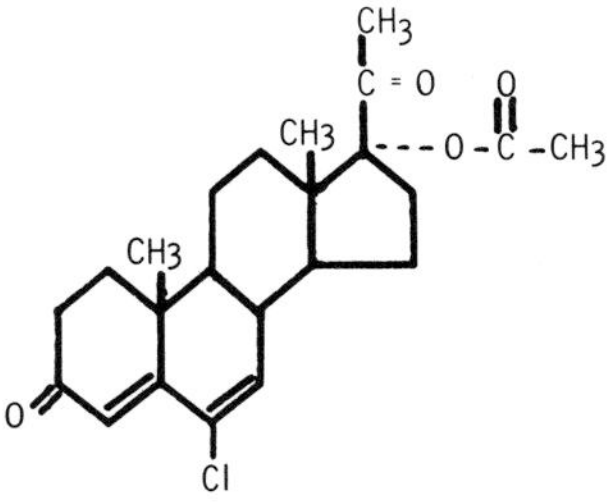

6 chloro - 6 dehydro - 17 – acetoxy
progesterone
(Chlormadinone)

Fig. 8-3. Pregnane derivatives with progestational activity. Note structural relationship to progesterone.

estrogens (Premarin®) and interposing small doses of ethisterone for three to five days at monthly intervals for a period of one year. One of the two cases presented in chart form in the original communication is shown in Table 8-1, and the history of this case is as follows:

Miss B., 21 years old, complained of passing endometrial casts with severe pain. A dilatation and curettage afforded no relief. It was decided to suppress ovulation by the continuous administration of estrogens, superimposing 10 mg of ethisterone three times a day for three consecutive days each month. After an intramuscular dose of 5 mg of estradiol dipropionate, the patient was immediately placed on conjugated estrogens (Premarin®), 1.25 mg four times a day for one month, three times a day for the second month, twice a day for the next seven months; then the dose was reduced to 1.25 mg once per day for the remaining three months of therapy. All estrogen therapy was discontinued about one year after the start. Ethisterone was continued at monthly intervals for two months afterward in order to avoid excessive breakthrough bleeding. Basal body temperature records were kept during therapy and all cycles appeared to be anovulatory without cast formation and painless.

Table 8-1. Treatment of membranous dysmenorrhea in a woman 21 years of age. Ovulation was suppressed for one year by the continuous administration of an estrogen in descending doses. An oral progestin was superimposed for three days each month to assure a withdrawal bleeding period. (Reproduced from Greenblatt, R. B., 1954, Am. J. Obst. & Gynec. 68: 835.)

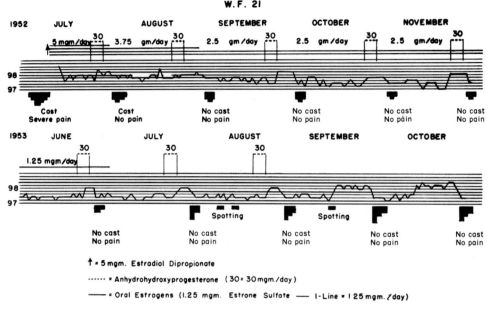

Comment. The management of patients with membranous dysmenorrhea by the continuous suppression of ovulation for a period of one year has proved not only simple in execution but also most gratifying to the patient. After discontinuation of therapy, ovulatory menses usually set in within a few months, and it has appeared that fertility was enhanced after the induced infertility. The administration of those antiovulatory agents which are potent progestational agents from day 5 to day 25 of the cycle is contraindicated in such patients, since cast formation is aggravated rather than eliminated.

Limitation of Fertility

Heretofore, most of the published data on antifertility studies have dealt with Enovid® (containing 9.85 mg of norethynodrel and 0.15 mg of ethinyl estradiol 3 methyl ether (EE3ME), administered once or more per day. Extensive studies have shown, however, that one-half of the above dosage was adequate. The interest of Greenblatt, et al. in this field has been concerned with much lower dosage, i. e. 2.5 mg of norethynodrel and 0.1 mg of EE3ME per day. The administration of this agent in this range has proved fairly satisfactory, although maintenance of the vascularity of the endometrium often proved inadequate and mild breakthrough bleeding made its appearance between the sixteenth and twenty-third day. When this phenomenon occurred, the dosage was raised for the remaining days with favorable results. The basal body temperature (BBT) record, to ascertain whether ovulation is inhibited, is useful only when nonthermogenic progestins are employed, such as 6-dehydro-retroprogesterone, or when the dose of norethynodrel is 2.5 mg or less.

A sufficient number of cases have been treated with this dosage so that certain conclusions are permissible, mainly that the repression of ovulation was the rule. Evidence favoring this conclusion was furnished by the BBT which in most instances remains depressed and uniphasic. In some cases there was a rise in BBT from the seventh or eighth day onward to the end of therapy. When this occurred the BBT could not be used to indicate whether ovulation took place. Marked decrease or absence of pregnanediol and lowering of urinary gonadotropins below 6 M. U. on day 21 of the cycle were laboratory tools that yielded confirmatory information. (Table 8-2). In most instances the ferning

Table 8-2. Physiologic effects of 2.5 mg norethynodrel with 0.1 mg EE3ME on basal temperature record, cervical mucus, endometrium, and Huhner test in a selected group of patients.

Patient	Basal temperature record day 5 - 25	Cervical mucus		Endometrium		Huhner test	
		14th d.	21st d.	14th d.	21st d.	14th d.	21st d.
M. W. * #	Uniphasic	Luteal	Luteal	E-Ps	M	Neg.	–
B. S. *	Uniphasic	Fern	Fern		M	Pos.	Pos.
C. B.	Thermogenic	Fern	–	E-Ps	M	–	–
J. R.	Thermogenic	–	Fern		P-	–	–
L. N. * #	Uniphasic	–	Fern		M	–	Pos.

* Urinary pregnanediol valures negative or minimal on day 21 of cycle
# Urinary gonadotrophins not detectable on day 21 of cycle
E-Ps = estrogenic with presecretory; M = mixed estrogenic and secretory;
P- = imperfect secretory

phenomenon of cervical mucus was not abolished, and the Sims-Huhner test showed good sperm motility throughout the cycle. Occasionally, the ferning ability of the cervical mucus was lost by the fourteenth day, but more constantly so when larger doses were administered. Sperm migration or survival in such mucus is very poor. Moreover, the endometrium at this dose range showed estrogenic effects with some presecretory or secretory changes on day 14 (Fig. 8-4). The proliferative glands persisted along with some secretory changes by day 21, so that a favorable nidus for ovum implantation was improbable (Fig. 8-5). When larger doses of antiovulatory agents were employed, excellent

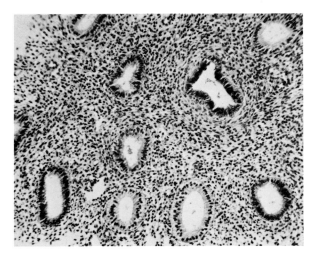

Fig. 8-4. Endometrial biopsy on 14th day of cycle in a patient receiving 2.5 mg of norethynodrel with 0.1 mg of 3 methyl ether of ethinyl estradiol from day 5 of the cycle. The basal temperature was elevated from day 7 and the cervical mucus was luteal. The endometrium shows a proliferative stage with some glands in the presecretory phase.

presecretory to secretory changes were already present by day 14, and by day 21 the endometrium frequently was in an advanced secretory state, or else the secretory glands were in a regressive stage with marked decidual changes. In either case, it is believed, such changes are inimical for ovum implantation.

Mention should be made that on rare occasions a withdrawal period does not follow antiovulatory therapy; this has been termed "silent menstruation" by Rock and his co-workers [25]. In such instances, medication should be resumed within eight days to avoid escape of ovulation. It should be stated that ovulation may not be inhibited if the antiovulatory agents are started as late as day 10 of the cycle. The incidence of nausea appeared to be less frequent the smaller the dose of estrogen employed. Tyler and Olson [28] found varying frequencies of occurrence of "reactions" with different antiovulatory compounds.

It should be emphasized that when an estrogen is administered with a progestogen for ovulation control, it is the estrogen that actually blocks ovulation. The progestational agent merely insures a constancy to the cycle by inducing withdrawal bleeding with regularity while in all probability enhancing the antiovulatory effect of the estrogen. Because of this belief, Greenblatt, et al. have administered from 0.05 to 0.1 mg of ethinyl estradiol from day 5 to day 19 of the cycle, followed by a

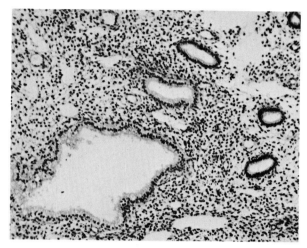

Fig. 8-5. Endometrial biopsy on the 21st day of cycle in a patient receiving 2.5 mg of norethynodrel with 0.1 mg of 3 methyl ether of ethinyl estradiol. The basal temperature was depressed and uniphasic, the cervical mucus was clear and watery and ferned on drying. The Sims-Huhner test was positive. The endometrium shows secretory changes with persistence of proliferative glands.

progestational agent such as 12.5 to 25 mg of dimethisterone from day 20 to 24 [2]. However, escape of ovulation occasionally occurred on this regimen, and the estrogen dosage has been extended to day 25 of the cycle with the progestogen added from day 21 to day 25. Experiences with 0.1 mg EE from day 5 to day 25, and 25 mg of dimethisterone added to the estrogen from day 21 to day 25, have been quite satisfactory.

Essential Dysmenorrhea

Wilson and Kurzrok [30] found that in the human being the maximal amplitude in uterine contractions occurred during the luteal phase and hence interdicted the use of progesterone. In clinical practice, however, progesterone administered during the last ten days of the cycle has proved beneficial in many cases, while in others it has increased the discomfort.

In recalcitrant cases, the cyclic inhibition of ovulation for a period of six to twelve months has afforded the patient a respite for a considerable period of time and not infrequently has proved curative. Such inhibition is best attained by the administration of a potent estrogen such as 0.1 mg EE or its equivalent from day 5 to day 25 of the cycle, along with a progestin from day 21 to day 25. When medication is stopped, ovulatory menstruation returns within one or two months, and frequently menses are painless for an unpredictable period of time [9]. Other methods for the suppression of ovulation for the relief of dysmenorrhea are available by simply administering antiovulatory drugs from day 5 to day 24 inclusive of the cycle, just as in the control of conception [29]. A brief case history follows:

Table 8-3 records the management of a young woman with severe essential dysmenorrhea. Conjugated estrogens (Premarin®), 5 mg daily from day 5 to day 24, were sufficient to suppress ovulation, and a painless menstrual period occurred on time. When a placebo was used in the same manner, the result was most unsatisfactory. That the administration of 2.5 mg of norethynodrel with 0.1 mg of EE3ME was followed by anovulatory periods may be judged by the absence of pregnanediol in the urine on day 21 of the cycle on two occasions, the persistence of ferning of the cervical mucus, and the satisfactory relief of pain. Larger doses of an antiovulatory agent may predispose towards decidual cast formation, and the passage of such a cast is frequently, but not always, associated with painful cramps.

Table 8-3. Successful treatment of dysmenorrhea by repression of ovulation in a white female aged 17 years. Medication was given from day 5 to day 24 inclusive of the cycle. Note that severe pain was experienced when a placebo was administered.

Patient	Course	Drug	Test	Results
1. Hunt w. f. 17	1	Premarin.® 5 mg. /day		Painless
	2	Placebo		Severe pain
	3	Norethynodrel 2.5 mg. with 0.1 mg. 3-Methyl ether of ethinyl estradiol	Pregnanediol 21st day = 0 mg.	Dosage increased 23rd day because of spotting. Period painless.
	4	"	Ferning 21st day	90% improvement
	5	"	Pregnanediol 21st day = 0 mg.	Painless period

Hypermenorrhea

Menorrhagia (functional uterine bleeding) is readily brought under control by the administration of adequate doses of progesterone with estrogen and/or androgen, or by the use of 20 to 40 mg of Norlutin® or Enovid® for a period of five to ten days. In contradistinction to menometrorrhagia, the management of hypermenorrhea, i.e. cyclic ovulatory menstruation that is excessive and prolonged, has proved far less satisfactory. Heretofore, androgens were administered during the last half of the cycle in the hope of lessening the amount of flow, or progestins were administered in the hope of inducing more rapid and complete desquamation of the endometrium. Both androgens and progestins proved helpful in about 50 per cent of the cases, as did toluidine blue (Blutene) in a few others who may have had some clotting defect. Many who did not respond to the above regimen fared much better when ovulation was suppressed by the administration of potent progestins such as Enovid®, Norlutin®, or Provera®, in combination with an estrogen, from day 5 to day 25 of the cycle. Rock [25] felt that excessive or prolonged menstruation could be restrained within acceptable limits in at least 75 per cent of cycles if ovulation were suppressed using the day 5 to 25 regimen of 10 to 20 mg of Enovid® or Norlutin®, daily.

Endometriosis

The utility of the continuous suppression of ovulation for periods of six months or longer by 19-norsteroids or estrogen and progestational compounds has been well established [1], [18]. The induction of pseudopregnancy has been shown to be beneficial in over 50 per cent of patients diagnosed as having endometriosis. The improvement was manifested not only by reduction of pain but by the disappearance of palpable painful ovarian masses, induration of the cul-de-sac, and uterosacral ligaments or obvious endometrial implants. After cessation of therapy, normal ovulatory menses return within one to three months and frequently without discomfort. If pelvic discomfort and dysmenorrhea return, a second or even a third course may be instituted. Table 8-4 records the progress of a patient who obtained excellent relief during

Table 8-4. Induction of pseudopregnancy with norethindrone in a white female aged 34 with endometriosis and severe pain for two weeks in each month.

Date	Medication, Results, Remarks	
Mar. 15/58	Norethindrone, 20 mg./day continuously.	Pelvic induration, pelvic mass
Nov. 7/58	Some spotting - increased dosage to 40 mg. per day for few days and then reduced to 30 mg./day until end of 9th month	Weight gain of 10 lbs. 90% improvement. Mild acne. Libido diminished
Dec. 15/58	Stopped Rx - two days later passed fragmented cast	Menses scanty but painful. Gained 20 pounds.
Jan. 6/59	Normal 3 day menses - 50% pain	Marked reduction in pelvic induration and mass.

a course of nine months of therapy. When pain and discomfort returned, a second course of 15 to 16 months yielded similarly good results (Table 8-5). After several months the patient returned with recurrence of her symptoms, and a third course of antiovulatory therapy was instituted.

Table 8-5. Same patient as depicted in Table 8-4 to whom dimethisterone with estrogen was given over 15 months.

10 mg/day*	0.2 mg./d EE3ME	7 days	Breakthrough bleeding on 7th day.
50 mg/day	1 mg./d EE3ME	5 days	Dosage increased to stop bleeding.
20 mg/day	0.2 mg./d EE3ME	2 mos.	Asymptomatic. Some spotting.
25 mg/day	0.2 mg./d EE3ME	2 mos.	Asymptomatic. Some spotting.
35 mg/day	0.09 mg./d EE3ME	2 mos.	Asymptomatic. Some spotting.
25 mg/day	0.3 mg./d EE3ME	9 mos.	Asymptomatic. No spotting. Pelvic mass gone. Felt well. No weight gain. Endometrial biopsy was secretory. Two months after cessation of medication, normal menses returned with mild pain

EE = Ethinyl Estradiol
EE3ME = Ethinyl Estradiol-3-Methyl Ether
*Dimethisterone ®

Unexplained Infertility

Where infertility is unexplained in that both members of a barren marriage are apparently normal, the "resting" or perhaps the "disturbing" of the pituitary-ovarian axis for a period of three to six months, by suppression of ovulation or by modifying pituitary activity, has been followed by conception in a surprisingly good number. Rock and his group [24] have reported that up to 20 to 30 per cent of such cases conceived within a few months after cessation of therapy. Although the incidence of success falls in the statistical norm for infertility couples, it should be recalled that this technique was tried in those patients in whom other methods had failed. The therapeutic test is often referred to as the Rock rebound phenomenon, although Rock himself disclaims any such pretensions for the method. The treatment is similar to that used for dysmenorrhea.

Mittelschmerz

Middle-of-the-month pain that coincides with the time of ovulation is known as mittelschmerz. This event may be associated with extreme pain and may prove incapacitating for a few days in each month. In many patients the appendix has been removed because the acute onset simulated acute appendicitis. The basal temperature record is extremely useful in diagnosis. Many women with this syndrome have suffered much at the hands of many physicians. In severe, recurring cases, the pain may be alleviated by the suppression of ovulation for several consecutive months. This may be accomplished by cyclic estrogen and progestin therapy as outlined in the treatment of essential dysmenorrhea (Table 8-6) or by the cyclic administration of antiovulatory drugs from day 5 to day 25 of the cycle. After a four- to six-month period of therapy, symptoms may not return. In others, recurrence of the syndrome necessitates further courses of therapy (Table 8-7).

Table 8-6. Treatment of mittelschmerz by inhibition of ovulation.

	Age	Estrogen d. 5-19	Dimethisterone d. 20-24	No. of cycles	BTR	Results
No. 1—R.	21	0.1 mg. EE	25 mg.	3	Anovulatory	Good
No. 2—M.	30	0.1 mg. EE	25 mg.	3	Anovulatory	Good
No. 3—L.J.	18	0.1 mg. EE	25 mg.	1	Anovulatory	Good
No. 4—O.	29	0.1 mg. EE	25 mg.	3	Anovulatory	Good
No. 5—V.	29	0.1 mg. EE	25 mg.	1	Anovulatory	Good

EE = Ethinyl Estradiol

Table 8-7. Treatment of mittelschmerz by administration of antiovulatory drugs from day 5 to day 25 of cycle.

Treatment	How administered	Remarks
1. Norlutin® 20-30 mg.	Continuously for 4 mos.	Excellent relief for 12 mos., then return of signs and symptoms
2. Norlutin Acetate 10 mg.	Day 5 - 25	Breakthrough bleeding on 17th day
3. Enovid® 20 mg.	Day 5 - 25 x 2 mos.	A little nausea first few days. Excellent relief #
4. Enovid® 10 mg.	Day 5 - 25 x 3 mos. *	Did not prevent mittelschmerz. Breakthrough bleeding third month of Rx.
5. Norethynodrel 5 mg. EE3ME 0.2 mg.	Day 5 - 25 x 4 mos.	Satisfactory
6. Enovid® 15 mg.	Day 5 - 25 x 3 mos.	Satisfactory
7. Enovid® 10 mg.	Day 5 - 25 x 2 mos.	Satisfactory #

*Emotionally upset.
#Return of syndrome without Rx

Premenstrual Tension

Progestogens have been used for the alleviation of the tension experienced by many women prior to the onset of menstruation ever since Israel [17] first recommended progesterone for seven to ten days before the onset of menses in 1948. However, there are those with such major menstrual molimina that more heroic measures are required to mitigate their distress. In these, inhibition of ovulation by the administration of Enovid® in 5 mg. doses from day 5 to day 24 inclusive has proved invaluable. Heller [16] reported that he successfully treated 20 patients for at least three menstrual cycles and felt that they would remain asymptomatic for upwards of six cycles. Good results have been obtained by inhibiting ovulation with 0.1 mg EE from day 5 to day 19, then giving a mild progestinal agent such as dimethisterone from day 20 to day 24 (Table 8-8) [2] .

Table 8-8. Treatment of premenstrual tension by inhibition of ovulation.

Patient	Age	Estrogen d. 5-19	Dimethis- terone® d. 20-24	No. of cycles	BTR	Results
No. 1–F. K.	30	0.1 mg. EE	25 mg.	3	Anovulatory	Good
No. 2–B. B.	37	0.1 mg. EE	25 mg.	10	Anovulatory	Good
No. 3–L. W.	28	0.1 mg. EE	25 mg.	15	Anovulatory	Very good, no weight gain
No. 4–K. G.	40	0.1 mg. EE	25 mg.	6	Anovulatory	Good
No. 5–G. L.	34	0.1 mg. EE	25 mg.	1	Anovulatory	Good
No. 6–C. –	16	0.1 mg. EE	25 mg.	1	Anovulatory	Good
No. 7–T.	23	0.5 mg. Estriol	20 mg.	1	Anovulatory	Good
No. 8–D. A.	39	0.1 mg. EE	25 mg.	6	Anovulatory	Fair
No. 9–S. H.	13	0.1 mg EE	25 mg.	1	Anovulatory	Fair
No. 10–E. H.	35	0.1 mg. EE	25 mg.	1	Anovulatory	Discontinued, nausea on EE
No. 11–D. Mc.	28	0.1 mg.	25 mg.	1	Anovulatory	Discontined, nausea on EE

EE = Ethinyl Estradiol

DISCUSSION

What antiovulatory agents are available and which are of practical value? Steroids existing in nature such as testosterone, progesterone, and estrone can inhibit ovulation in women [5]. Practically, however, testosterone and other androgens are undesirable because of the side effects produced. Progesterone and many so-called pure progestational substances require very large doses, and their actions are too variable and the occurrence of breakthrough bleeding too frequent. Estrogens are the most effective inhibitors, but escape of ovulation occurs in the succeeding cycle unless medication is very precisely employed or administered continuously. Other agents have been used experimentally, such as the administration of gonadotropic hormones of animal origin which, after a given time, produce antigonadotropins. The unpredictability of duration of effect and the inherent difficulties of the methods preclude their use.

The most potent oral ovulation inhibitors are certain 19-norsteroids either having both estrogenic and progestational activity or being capable of at least partial conversion to estrogen *in vivo*. Enovid® (norethynodrel with 3 methyl ether of ethinyl estradiol), Norlutin® (norethindrone), and Norlutate® with EE (norethindrone acetate with ethinyl estradiol), as well as other potent progestins such as Provera®, when combined with an adequate estrogen, have proved most useful and practical antiovulatory agents. Enovid® in 5 mg doses has been subjected to wide clinical study with the finding that ovulation can be successfully inhibited in succeeding cycles over a period of years without harmful effects if administered from day 5 to day 24 inclusive in each cycle [20], [21].

Relatively low doses of oral estrogens are effective blockers of ovulation in women. The cyclic oral estrogen administration alone from day 5 to day 25 yields unpredictable withdrawal periods both as to time of withdrawal and amount and length of flow. However, if a progestin is added from day 21 to day 25, a uniformity in cyclic bleeding is assured, and in a limited trial the results were promising. Moreover, the continuous rather than cyclic administration of an estrogen, but with an oral progestational agent superimposed at monthly intervals for several days, was shown to be effective in repressing ovulation for as much as one year at a time [9], [14]. Whether such a method is ideal or not may be open to question. It is nevertheless of some historic interest in that it anticipated the antifertility era by demonstrating blocking of ovulation for long periods of time without harm.

SUMMARY

Antiovulatory agents have proved of clinical value in the management of severe mittelschmerz, essential dysmenorrhea, membranous dysmenorrhea, endometriosis, hypermenorrhea, and premenstrual tension, as well as in the control of conception.

REFERENCES

1. Andrews, M.C., Andrews, W.C., and Straus, A.F. 1959. *Am. J. Obstet. & Gynec.* 78: 776.
2. Aydar, C.K., and Greenblatt, R.B. 1961. *J. Med. Assn. State of Alabama* (Sept.) 31.
3. Cook, H.H., Gamble, C.J., and Satterthwaite, A.P. 1961. *Am. J. Obstet. & Gynec.* 82: 437.
4. Dominguez, H., Simotitz, F., and Greenblatt, R.B. *Am. J. Obstet. & Gynec.*
5. Drill, V. 1959. *Proc. 6th Internat. Conf. on Planned Parenthood,* New Delhi, India, Feb., 16.
6. Garcia, C.R., Pincus, G., and Rock, J. 1958. *Am. J. Obstet. & Gynec.* 75: 82.
7. Goldzieher, J., Moses, L.E., and Ellis, L.T. 1962. *J.A.M.A.* 180 (May 5): 359.
8. Greenblatt, R.B. 1961. *Med. Clin. North America* 45: 973 (July).
9. Greenblatt, R.B. 1952. *Office Endocrinology,* Chap. 28, C.C. Thomas, Springfield, Ill.
10. Greenblatt, R.B. 1961. *Proc. III Weltkongress fur Gynak und Geburts* (Vienna) vom. 3.9 - 9.9.
11. Greenblatt, R.B., 1962. *Excerpta Medica* No. 51, Internat. Cong. on Hormonal Steroids (Milan), May 14-19, Abstr. 274, 204.
12. Greenblatt, R.B., 1959. *Proc. of Sympos. on Enovid,* Searle Res. Labs., Chicago, 4-10.
13. Greenblatt, R.B., and Barfield, W.E. 1959. *South. Med. J.* 52: 345.
14. Greenblatt, R.B., Hammond, D.O., and Clark, S.L. 1954. *Am. J. Obstet. & Gynec.* 68: 835.
15. Greenblatt, R.B., and Jungck, E.C. 1958. *J.A.M.A.* 166: 1461 (Mar. 22).
16. Heller, C.G., 1956. *Int. Rec. Med.* 169: 760.
17. Israel, S.L. 1938. *J.A.M.A.* 110: 1721.
18. Kistner, R.W. 1959. *Clin. Obstet. & Gynec.* 2: 877.
19. Pincus, G., Rock, J., Garcia, C.R., Rice-Wray, E., Paniagua, M., and Rodriguez, I. 1958. *Am. J. Obstet. & Gynec.* 75: 1333.
20. Pincus, G. 1960. *Proc. 1st Internat. Congr. Endocrinol.* Copenhagen, Denmark, July, 138.
21. Pincus, G., Garcia, C.R., Rock, J., and others. 1959. *Science* 130 (July 10): 81.
22. Rice-Wray, E. 1957. Proc. of Sympos. on 19-Nor Progestational Steroids, Searle Res. Labs. Chicago, 75-88.

23. Rice-Wray, E., Schulz-Contreras, M., Guerrero, I., and Aranda-Rosell, A. 1962. *J. A. M. A.* 180 (May 5): 355.
24. Rock, J., Garcia, C. R., and Pincus, G. 1957. *Recent Progress in Hormone Research,* Academic Press, New York.
25. Rock, J., Garcia, C. R., and Pincus, G. 1960. *Am. J. Obstet. & Gynec.* 79: 758.
26. Sturgis, S. H., and Albright, F. 1940. *Endocrinology* 26: 68.
27. Tyler, E. T.
28. Tyler, E. T., and Olsen, H. J. 1959. *J. A. M. A.* 169: 1843.
29. Weinberg, C. H. 1959. *Proc. of Sympos. on Enovid,* Part II, Searle Res. Labs. Chicago, 50: 7.
30. Wilson, L., and Kurzrok, R. 1940. *Endocrinology* 27: 23.

IX

Robert B. Greenblatt, M.D., C.M.
FUNCTIONAL UTERINE BLEEDING

INTRODUCTION

Functional uterine bleeding, once the dismay of the gynecologist, may now be brought readily under control. With a better understanding of the physiopathology of the ovarian-uterine axis and the advent of new potent progestational agents, the problem should no longer prove baffling to the physician nor a scourge to suffering womankind.

The clinician not oriented along the lines of glandular physiology will resort to repeated curettage, hysterectomy, or radiation therapy. How many young women have had half a dozen or more currettements only to end up with a hysterectomy? How frequently have young nulliparous women been subjected to radiation therapy only to become gynecologic cripples thereafter? Admittedly, there is a place and time for such methods, but often these measures are undertaken by the clinician as a matter of expediency or because of failure to familiarize himself with the advantages of various hormonal measures [3], [4], [12], [15], [19]. In the past, the purported causes of uterine bleeding were frequently fantastic. Early in the 19th century, Gardien bitterly blamed "cette danse voluptueuse sous le nom de Walse." It is amusing to recall the causes of uterine hemorrhage as listed by Dewees in his *Treatise on Diseases of the Female* published in 1837. "Women," he wrote, "are most obnoxious to menorrhagia

who live indolently and indulge in stimuli
who use little or no exercise
who keep late hours
who dance inordinately
who are intemperate
who have borne many children
who have been subject to febrile affections
who have much leucorrhea
who are too prodigal of the joys of wedlock

142

who are advancing toward the non-menstrual period
who yield too readily to passions or emotions of the mind."

Save for recent times, the annals of gynecology are filled with pages of blundering concepts and primitive practices in the management of functional uterine bleeding. In fact, gynecologists may not look back with any degree of pride on the methods in vogue in past years and employed even to this day in combatting excessive uterine bleeding. The Hippocratic concept of "fluor albus" and "fluor rubor" jogged uneventfully along, and even the Renaissance in medicine experienced at the end of the last century and the beginning of this one failed to add much in treatment that would change the age-old usage of cooling the abdomen and raising the foot of the bed. It is true that to ergot therapy other agents have been added in the therapeutic armamentarium, such as calcium, snake venom, and vitamin preparations. Curettage of a crude form was introduced in Roman times, but whether it was used in uterine bleeding is conjectural. This much is certain; that the universal use of the curette today, particularly in the treatment of menorrhagia of adolescent girls, is an admission that simple physiologic principles as to the causes of this functional disorder remain misunderstood. Moreover, hysterectomy and radiation therapy have gained an unwarranted foothold in therapy [17]. All this, simply because the lessons to be learned from the study of the physiology of menstruation are not properly applied.

Functional uterine bleeding has been defined as abnormal and excessive bleeding that occurs because of physiologic disturbances and not pathologic processes. Hormonal dysfunction is the principal cause, but nutritional, nervous, and psychogenic factors also play important roles. Bleeding associated with pathologic lesions, such as endometrial polyps, pelvic inflammatory disease, endometriosis, and, to a great extent, fibromyomas of the uterus, may also be brought under control in a manner similar to that employed in purely functional disorders. This does not imply that endometriosis or fibromyomas disappear as a result of therapy, but only that hemostasis is induced. With but few exceptions, however, bleeding associated with underlying pathology does not and cannot be expected to respond to hormonal therapy. Included in the category of organic causes for bleeding are cervical polyps, cervical carcinoma, uterine malignancies, carcinoma of the Fallopian tubes, ectopic pregnancy, misconceptions, and blood dyscrasias. Bleeding from uteri with submucous fibromyomas or large endometrial polyps, or from uteri previously subjected to radiation therapy, usually proves refractory to endocrine therapy [9].

Many physicians, having employed glandular therapy in a haphazard and reckless manner and finding it wanting, decry its use. Others refuse to try hormones, asserting that their employment is experimental or that they are carcinogenic. To assert that several planned courses of estrogens are carcinogenic is as unjust as it is unfounded.

The concept of a relationship of estrogens to cancer is a prejudice retained as a result of experiments performed more than three decades ago by Lacassagne on a cancer strain of mice. That this simple relationship does not hold for most other laboratory animals or for infrahuman forms such as the macaque seems to have been overlooked. Furthermore, the incidence of deaths from breast and uterine cancer as reported from the state of Massachusetts has not changed significantly in the last 30 years in spite of the universal use and abuse of hormones [20].

The problem of uterine bleeding should be approached with caution and reservation, for the foremost duty of the physician is to rule out malignancy as the cause. A curettage and cervical biopsies will usually rule out endometrial and cervical carcinoma. Curettage will prove therapeutically effective where retained products of conception or cervical or endometrial polyps are present, and will be remedial in 50 to 60 per cent of the patients with functional uterine bleeding. The questions which arise are: What is to be the approach in the management of the patient who does not improve following curettage, or whose improvement is temporary and fleeting? What is the role of radical surgery and radiation therapy in such instances? What is the place of hormonal therapy in the scheme?

The knowledge gained from the study of the physiology of menstruation may be applied most effectively in the treatment of menstrual disorders. At the risk of oversimplification, it may be stated that normal menstruation occurs as a result of rather rapid withdrawal of hormonal support (estrogen and progesterone) of the endometrium, with consequent shedding of the endometrium (Fig. 9-1). In anovulatory menstruation, estrogen only is withdrawn, with the result that shedding is gradual and incomplete, and quite frequently the bleeding may be excessive and prolonged (Fig. 9-2). Menstrual bleeding stops, it is believed, when the functionally renewable layers of the endometrium have been more or less completely shed. Shedding may be irregular and incomplete at times, even in patients with ovulatory menstruation, resulting in cyclic hypermenorrhea. It has been suggested that this is due to improper metabolism of progesterone or to faulty regression of the corpus luteum. On the other hand, ultra-complete shedding may occur, as in the passage of a decidual cast of the uterus. This is thought to be a hyperprogestational effect, and though it is most often attended by scant bleeding, occasionally there is excessive bleeding and severe pain [13].

It has been shown that in the castrate monkey, estrogen deprivation bleeding may be postponed by administering progesterone as soon as estrogens are discontinued. Engle, et al. [6] have demonstrated that progesterone has the power to suppress estrogen-deprivation bleeding. Furthermore, Hisaw, Corner and others were able to prove that small doses of progesterone, administered for four or five consecutive days, will set off menstruation-like bleeding in castrated monkeys which continue to receive chronic doses of estrogen. It is of further interest to note that Zuckerman has shown that testosterone behaves like estrogen or progesterone in that it may postpone estrogen withdrawal bleeding [2], [5], [6], [14], [22]. Furthermore, it has been demonstrated that progesterone will postpone estrogen-withdrawal bleeding, but that neither estrogen nor testosterone in physiologic doses will prevent progesterone-withdrawal bleeding (Figs. 9-3 and 9-4). Albeit, estrogens in very large doses (sometimes astronomic) may arrest progesterone withdrawal bleeding.

Ovulatory Menstruation

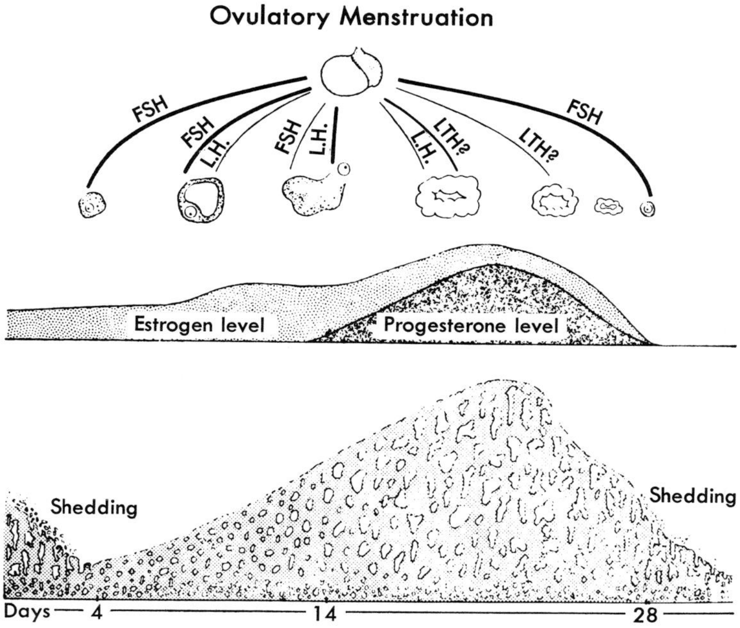

Fig. 9-1. Pituitary-ovarian-endometrial relationships in normal ovulation. (Reproduced from Greenblatt, R.B., 1952, *Office Endocrinology*, C.C Thomas, Springfield, Ill.)

Experience with the use of gonadal steroids in the therapy of various gynecic disorders has crystallized sufficiently to warrant certain categorical statements insofar as they pertain to the phenomenon of uterine bleeding [10].

ESTROGENS

Uterine bleeding may be brought on by a sudden lowering of estrogen levels (estrogen-deprivation bleeding). Breakthrough bleeding

Anovulatory Bleeding

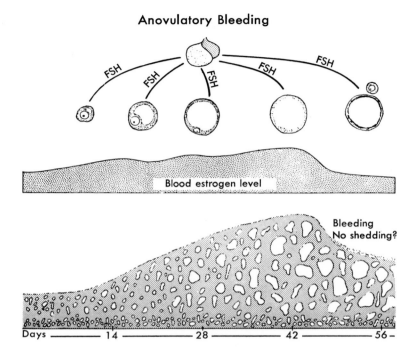

Fig. 9-2. Pituitary-ovarian-endometrial relationships in anovulatory bleeding. (Reproduced - *Ibid.*, Fig. 9-1).

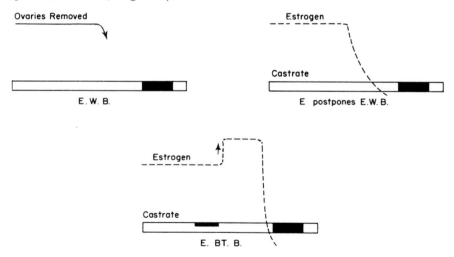

E.W.B. = Estrogen withdrawal bleeding
E. BT. B. = Estrogen breakthrough bleeding

Fig. 9-3. Estrogen-withdrawal bleeding in the macaque. Experiments of Edgar Allen, George W. Corner, and others. (Reproduced from Greenblatt, R.B., 1959, *Clinical Obst. & Gynec.* 2: 232.)

will result from constant and prolonged estrogen stimulation. In
either case, the administration of sufficiently large doses of estrogens
will raise the estrogen levels and usually bleeding will be arrested.
Parenteral estrogen, followed by descending oral doses, may be used
to good advantage. More rapid hemostasis may be obtained by the intravenous use of conjugated estrogens (Premarin®, Intravenous). The
dosage is 20 mg given intravenously every four to eight hours until
bleeding is arrested. Then oral estrogen therapy such as conjugated
estrogens (Premarin®) or the equivalent, in doses of 3.75 mg per day,
gradually reduced to 1.25 mg per day, is given for a period of three
weeks (Fig. 9-5). Then a progestin such as 5 mg of Norlutin®, Enovid®,
Provera®, or their equivalents, is administered for five days. A withdrawal period which will simulate a menstrual period will follow several
days later.

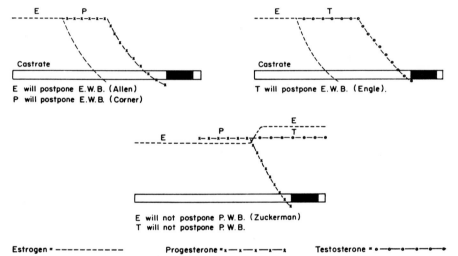

E will postpone E.W.B. (Allen)
P will postpone E.W.B. (Corner)

T will postpone E.W.B. (Engle).

E will not postpone P.W.B. (Zuckerman)
T will not postpone P.W.B.

Estrogen = ------------   Progesterone = ı—ı—ı—ı—ı   Testosterone = •—•—•—•—•—•

Fig. 9-4. The effect of progesterone or testosterone, which will postpone estrogen-withdrawal bleeding. Bleeding will occur after discontinuing a course
of progesterone in spite of continued estrogen or androgen treatment. (Reproduced - *Ibid.*, Fig. 9-3).

Estrogen therapy is particularly useful in the management of
functional uterine bleeding that occurs at the menarche and at the menopause. A complication of high dosage-estrogen therapy is nausea. The
errors that are most frequently made when employing estrogens are
the use of inadequate dosages and the abrupt cessation of therapy when
bleeding is arrested. Estrogens should be tapered off gradually.

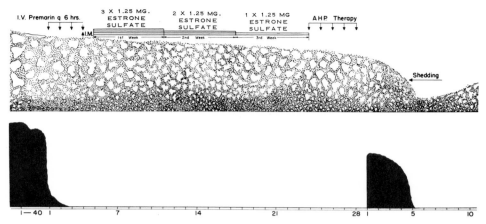

Fig. 9-5. Intravenous estrogens for the arrest of uterine bleeding. Bleeding is rapidly arrested if 20 mg of Premarin®(I.V.) is administered intravenously every four to six hours for two to four doses followed by an intramuscular injection of 20 mg. Premarin®(I.V.) and oral therapy is begun as follows: estrone sulfate tablets, 1.25 mg (or its equivalent) one t.i.d. for the first week, one b.i.d. for the second week, one daily for the third week, after which tablets of ethisterone, 30 mg per day (or its equivalent) are administered for five days. A normal withdrawal period usually follows. This method is preferable in adolescent cases and in those patients in whom it is desirable to delay the withdrawal period for at least one month. (Reproduced from Greenblatt, R.B., 1954, Med. Ann. Dist. of Columbia 23:187.

ANDROGENS

Androgens are not too effective in arresting a siege of uterine hemorrhage, but have proved useful in limiting the amount of bleeding and, more particularly, in preventing an ensuing bout of excessive bleeding as in patients with cyclic hypermenorrhea. Large doses of androgens (300 to 500 mg) over a short period of time, though not recommended, have, in some instances, proved capable of stopping severe bleeding. It is believed that androgens are myotonic and their effectiveness is thought to be due to the stimulating action on myometrial elements. Androgens per se are by no means the hormones of choice in the therapy of functional uterine bleeding. However, their value in patients who have excessive bleeding associated with fibromyomas, adenomyosis, or endometriosis cannot be denied. Clinicians using androgens alone to control bleeding will be disappointed in results in most cases. Furthermore, if high prolonged dosage is given, signs of virilization may be expected.

PROGESTOGENS

Prolonged bleeding is sometimes associated with faulty regression of the corpus luteum. In such instances, endometrial shedding may be incomplete, and consequently bleeding continues [16]. Progesterone is effective in postponing estrogen-deprivation and progesterone-deprivation bleeding, as well as progesterone breakthrough bleeding. Progesterone is a desquamative hormone. It increases the desquamation of vaginal epithelia and promotes the desquamation and shedding of the endometrium. Progesterone, as first pointed out by Albright [1], induces a "medical curettage."

Progesterone, when used parenterally in small doses (10 mg per day for five days) in the treatment of functional uterine bleeding, does not stop bleeding immediately though it may lessen it. Moreover, three to five days after the cessation of such a course of progesterone, bleeding may be considerably accentuated, though it stops finally about the seventh or eighth day after cessation of therapy. It was this accentuation of bleeding which probably led many of the earlier investigators to believe that progesterone was contraindicated in the treatment of bleeding.

The physiologic actions of progesterone seem to be paradoxical. Progesterone may be used to induce bleeding; it may be used to arrest bleeding. A better understanding of the physiologic properties of progesterone will result if the modus operandi of this hormone is explained in both amenorrhea and menorrhagia.

The amenorrheic female may or may not be producing adequate endogenous estrogens. If not (the vaginal cytology should reveal a hypoestrogenic smear), estrogen priming is necessary before progesterone will prove effective. In the amenorrheic female with adequate endogenous estrogens the following results may be expected when an oral progestational substance is administered (Fig. 9-6):

The administration of a progestational agent of low potency (1) daily for five days to an amenorrheic female with adequate endogenous estrogens frequently results in breakthrough bleeding before treatment is completed. However, if the same patient is treated with this same progestational agent, but with a higher dosage (2), bleeding will not occur until 24 to 72 hours after the cessation of the medication. If the same dosage is continued for ten days or longer, breakthrough bleeding often occurs before the tenth day (3). On the other hand, if the dosage is raised to a still much higher level (4), the medication may be continued for 30 days or longer without breakthrough bleeding.

It appears then that breakthrough bleeding will occur when inadequate amounts of progesterone are administered, but when adequate amounts are given, bleeding will be withheld until medication is withdrawn.

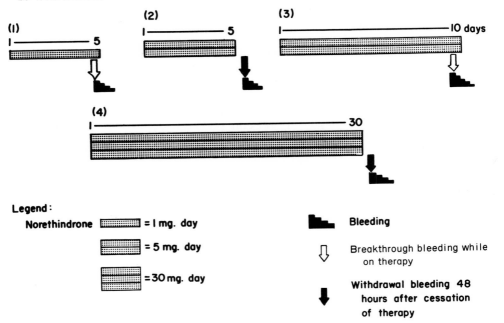

Fig. 9-6.　Amenorrheic female with adequate endogenous estrogens.　Progesterone and progestational agents may be employed to induce bleeding or to arrest bleeding. Some idea as to the physiologic actions of progestational substances in the amenorrheic female was afforded by the experiment outlined here.　Norethindrone, in varying doses of 1 mg, 5 mg, and 30 mg, was the progestational agent used.　(Reproduced - *Ibid.* Fig. 9-3).

The experience gained over the past fifteen years in the management of functional uterine bleeding is summarized in Fig. 9-7:

When 10 mg of progesterone are administered intramuscularly once daily for five consecutive days (A) to patients with functional uterine bleeding, bleeding does not stop, as a rule, but one to three days later the amount of bleeding increases and then it stops within five or six days—so that, all in all, twelve to fourteen days are required to arrest a bout of functional uterine bleeding on this dosage schedule.

If a single dose of 50 mg of progesterone is administered intramuscularly (B), bleeding will slow down considerably, and a few days later will increase in amount and continue for five to eight days, then stop.　Here again, ten to 12 days are required to arrest a bout of bleeding.

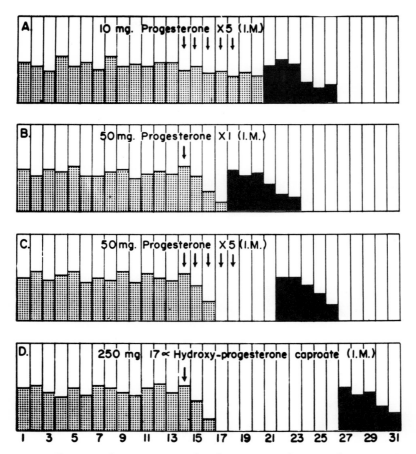

Fig. 9-7. Influence of progestational substance on functional uterine bleeding. (Reproduced - *Ibid*. Fig. 9-3).

If 50 mg of progesterone are administered intramuscularly once daily for five consecutive days (C), bleeding is frequently arrested within the first 48 hours of therapy, and a bleeding-free interval follows until two or three days after the last injection when a withdrawal period occurs which may last from five to seven days. In this way, the patient is afforded a bleeding-free interval of several days before onset of the withdrawal period.

When a single dose of 250 mg of 17 α-hydroxyprogesterone caproate is administered intramuscularly (D), bleeding is frequently arrested with 48 to 72 hours, and a bleeding-free interval of seven to ten days follows. A withdrawal period then occurs which lasts about five days, although it may be prolonged eight to nine days.

When using progestational agents in the treatment of functional uterine bleeding, it must be appreciated that progesterone in adequate doses will slow down and stop uterine bleeding, but that two to ten days after the progestational agent is withdrawn a withdrawal bleeding period will invariably follow—the length of time before occurrence of the withdrawal period depending on the nature of the progestational agent used.

The addition of estrogen and/or testosterone (both of which possess hemostatic properties) to 25 mg of progesterone enhances the effectiveness of progesterone, and bleeding will frequently stop within six to 24 hours after administration of this combination (Lukestra®, Sharp and Dohme; Tristerone®, Wyeth). If this combined hormone therapy is continued for five or six days, a withdrawal bleeding period of four to eight days will take place a few days after cessation of therapy. This has been previously described by the author as "arrest of bleeding according to plan" (Fig. 9-8).

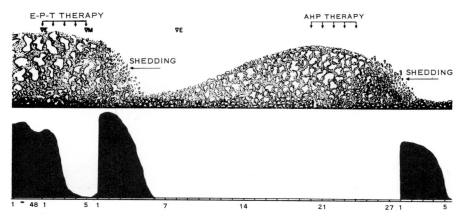

Fig. 9-8. The "arrest of bleeding according to plan." Practically every patient with uterine bleeding, excepting that due to misconceptions, blood dyscrasias, and malignant neoplasms, will respond to a therapeutic regimen known as "arrest of bleeding according to plan." This consists of 1.66 mg of estradiol benzoate or its equivalent, 25 mg of progesterone, and 25 mg of testosterone propionate, which are given for five to six consecutive days. Bleeding will stop within six to 36 hours and withdrawal bleeding will follow about 48 hours after cessation of therapy; this should simulate a normal mensis. Ethisterone (AHP)(30 mg per day for five days) or its equivalent should then be given from the 21st to the 25th days of the new cycle to prevent a recurrence of prolonged hemorrhage. (Reproduced - *Ibid.* - Fig. 9-3).

The errors attending the administration of progesterone are many. For example, physicians mistake the withdrawal period as a recurrence of the bleeding, and complicate the picture by immediately giving more progesterone. Another error frequently encountered is the cessation of therapy after only one or two days of progesterone medication because the bleeding was arrested. When free progesterone is used alone or in combination with other steroids, it is advisable to continue therapy for at least five days, even though bleeding may be arrested after the first day of therapy.

Two other points should be emphasized. First, whenever progesterone is employed, progesterone-withdrawal bleeding should be expected. The patient must be warned accordingly or she will feel that the therapy has failed. Second, a period of amenorrhea sets in after the progesterone-withdrawal bleeding, regardless of the method employed, and, in order to avoid a recurrence of hemorrhage, planned monthly courses of one of the progestational substances should be instituted to induce bleeding at cyclic monthly intervals. This cyclic therapy may be given each month for three to five months or longer until the patient resumes normal cyclic menstruation. This may be readily ascertained when the basal temperature record indicates that ovulation is occurring in a more or less regular manner [9] (Fig. 9-9).

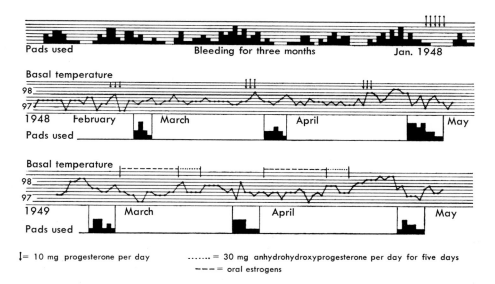

Fig. 9-9. Management of functional uterine bleeding in a 14-year-old girl who bled off and on since menarche at age 13. (Reproduced from [9a].)

Cyclic therapy may be given as follows: About 21 days after the *start* of the withdrawal bleeding period, one of the progestogens is administered daily for five consecutive days: ethisterone, 25 mg

(Lutocylol®, Ciba; Pranone®, Schering); 6α-methyl-17α-acetoxypro-
gesterone, 5 mg (Provera®, Upjohn); norethindrone, 5 mg (Norlutin®);
norethinodrel, 5 mg (Enovid®, Searle). Should the withdrawal bleeding be excessive during the first few days after administration of one
of the above, ergotrate (1/320th grain - 0.2 mg) may be given orally
every four to six hours for a total of four to six doses.

The intramuscular injection of progesterone in large doses is
often attended by pain or a local tissue reaction, and few patients will
tolerate more than 50 mg injected at any one site. Fortunately, many
of the handicaps associated with progesterone therapy in the past may
now be circumvented because of the availability of new groups of progestational agents:

Progesterone Derivatives

A single intramuscular dose of 250 mg of 17α-hydroxyprogesterone
caproate (Delalutin®, Squibb) will frequently arrest bleeding within
24 to 48 hours. Withdrawal bleeding will be postponed for seven to ten
days [7]. The administration of this long-acting progesterone in this
manner affords the patient a real breathing spell before withdrawal
bleeding occurs. The addition of a long-acting estrogen (Delestrogen®,
Squibb) enhances the effectiveness of 17α-hydroxyprogesterone caproate,
arresting bleeding in six to 24 hours.

The enhancing effect of estrogens on progesterone effectiveness
was demonstrated in this manner: When 125 mg of 17α-hydroxypro-
gesterone caproate was administered continuously twice weekly from
day 21 of a normal cycle, menses could be delayed for seven to ten
days. However, if 2.5 mg of estradiol valerate were added to this
progestational substance and given in the same manner, the normal
menstrual period could be postponed for several weeks or months.
Thus, these agents were capable of simulating to a great measure the
activity of the corpus luteum.

Substituted Progestogens for Oral Use

The 19-nortestosterone derivatives, norethindrone (Norlutin®)
and norethinodrel (Enovid®) for oral use are very potent progestational agents. In fact, norethindrone is not unlike the progesterone-
estrogen-androgen mixture previously recommended for the "arrest
of bleeding according to plan," for this potent progestational agent
has inherent estrogenic and androgenic propensities. Thirty milligrams orally (this dose may be doubled the first day in those instances
where loss of blood is heavy) will arrest functional uterine bleeding
within 24 hours in almost every instance. The medication is then continued in a dose of 15 to 30 mg daily for as long a period as desired,
usually until the hemoglobin has been restored toward normalcy. Withdrawal bleeding may thus be postponed for ten, 30, 90 days or longer,

as suits the patient and physician. Cyclic progestogens are then administered at monthly intervals. In many cases, cyclic therapy will
be needed for only five days in each month. In other instances, it may
be employed for 10 to 20 days each month if intermenstrual bleeding
occurs [12] (Fig. 9-10). In a few cases, because of heavy prolonged
withdrawal bleeding, pseudopregnancy for a period of many months has
been induced to the advantage of the patient [11].

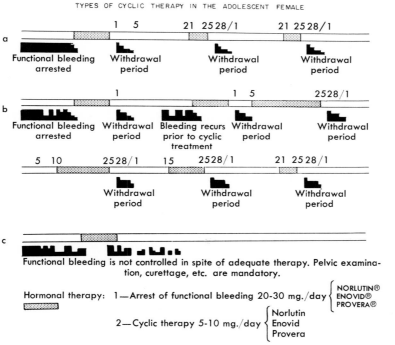

Fig. 9-10.   Pattern of hormone administration and responses in management of
functional uterine bleeding. (Reproduced from [12].)

HEMATOLOGIC FACTORS

Functional uterine bleeding occurs in adolescent girls and women
with iron-deficiency anemia [21]. The response to iron medication is
fairly rapid. Iron-deficiency anemia should not be mistaken for the
secondary anemia consequent to prolonged bleeding. However, iron
medication is indicated in all patients who have a low hemoglobin value.
The clotting time of the blood may be prolonged in girls who have
hypermenorrhea [18]. The excessive bleeding may or may not be from

an ovulatory endometrium. The administration of toluidine blue (Blutene chloride), 100 mg twice a day, is frequently attended by a significant reduction in blood loss.

Whenever menorrhagia is unresponsive to ordinary measures, a search should be made to detect blood dyscrasias such as aplastic anemia, leukemia, or thrombocytopenia. Idiopathic thrombopenic purpura often remains latent, and bleeding accompanying this condition may respond to progesterone therapy. In the course of time, however, the bleeding becomes more troublesome and the diagnosis should be suspected [8].

ADJUNCTIVE THERAPY

Adjunctive therapy must not be overlooked. Thyroid should be administered to those patients with evidence of hypothyroidism. Correction of body weight in the obese or undernourished and correction of dietary discrepancies must be a part of the regimen.

Attention should be given to the correction of unhappy environmental situations and to the removal of personality scars by appropriate psychotherapy. Bleeding in some instances is due to psychic maladjustment. A prolonged bout of bleeding has been observed following fright or some calamity such as the death of a member of the family. Psychosomatic disturbances play a greater role in menometrorrhagia than we have been wont to give credit. An inkling of such cause and effect is suggested by a passage from Luke concerning the woman who had bled for 12 years and who avowed she was cured after touching the border of Jesus' raiment. Jesus said to her, "Daughter, be of good comfort, thy faith hath made thee whole."

At least one dilatation and curettage is advisable in all adult women to rule out neoplasia before resorting to endocrine therapy. When a simple curettage fails to correct the disorder and when adequate hormonal trials have proved futile, then one may resort to hysterectomy. In menopausal and postmenopausal bleeding, radiation thereapy may be used only after thorough curettage has ruled out malignancy. In bleeding of the adolescent girl, radiation therapy is to be deprecated; curettage is rarely necessary and should be reserved for the very occasional instance when hormonal therapy fails to bring the uterine bleeding under control.

The management of a patient with functional uterine bleeding is frequently disconcerting and unsatisfactory because physician and patient expect permanent results to follow the employment of a single course of hormonal or other pharmacologic agents. It must be understood that the primary arrest of bleeding by such means is but a stop-gap mechanism without assurance against recurrence. However, the bleeding-free interval which follows affords an opportunity to correct the underlying causes of the disturbance. Subsequent planned therapy, continued for a sufficient length of time, will bring about cyclic menstruation with attendant ovulation in the greater number of patients. This is especially true in girls and young women, in whom salvage of reproductive powers is of prime importance.

The specter of cancer in association with uterine hemorrhagic disease is frightening. Great benefits will come to the patient by the assurance of the physician that malignancy has been ruled out. It is the office of the physician to inspire confidence of success, to calm and to comfort. This is a way of preparing the patient for endocrinotherapy, by lessening some of the influences which have set up disturbances in the hypothalamico-pituitary mechanism. Endocrinotherapy will prove of most value in the correction of the underlying disorder when the patient is placed in a receptive state.

Of the progestinal agents, norethindrone (Norlutin®) appears to be the most effective single hormonal preparation available for control of functional uterine bleeding. With its proper use in adequate dosage, bleeding may be and can be effectively controlled. Surgery and radiation therapy should be reserved for patients nearing the menopause or past their reproductive period.

CONCLUSIONS

This chapter, while bringing into broader view the advantages and limitations of hormonal measures, also summarizes the role of each of the steroids used in the control of functional uterine bleeding.

A plea is made to extend the long-accepted definition of the term "*functional* uterine bleeding" so that more women may receive the benefits of thoughtfully planned glandular therapy.

An attempt is made to divert the clinician from haphazard endocrine therapy as much as from reckless surgery.

In the management of dysfunctional bleeding, attention should be paid to several specific points.
1. Iron-deficiency anemia may be associated with prolonged bleeding, and iron replacement itself may be attended by rapid cessation of bleeding.
2. Emotional conflicts and stressful situations may contribute to the hypothalamico-pituitary-ovarian imbalance. Attempts should be made to correct underlying psychogenic problems, at the same time encouraging the patient to feel confident of success.
3. Parenteral progesterone with adequate estrogen and/or androgen, has proved most useful in control of functional uterine bleeding. The 19-norsteroids with added estrogens such as Norlutin® and Enovid®, have proved exceptionally valuable. Provera® with ethinyl estradiol, chlormadinone with ethinyl estradiol, and other progestins with estrogen may be employed orally to good advantage.

REFERENCES

1. Albright, F. 1938. *J. Maine M.A.* 29: 235.
2. Allen, E. 1927. Carnegie Inst. Washington, Publ. No. 380, *Contrib. Embryol.* No. 98, 29: 1.
3. Allen, W. M., and Heckel, G. P. 1942. *Am. J. Obstet. & Gynec.* 44: 984.
4. Browne, J. S. L. 1938. *Canad. M.A.J.* 39: 84.
5. Corner, G. W. 1942. *The Hormones in Human Reproduction,* Princeton Univ. Press, Princeton, Princeton, N. J.
6. Engle, E. T., Smith, P. E., and Shelesnyak, M. C. 1935. *Am. J. Obstet. & Gynec.* 29: 787.
7. Finkler, R. S. 1957. *Fertil. & Steril.* 8: 323.
8. Goldburgh, H. L., and Gouley, B. A. 1940. *Am. J. M. Sci.* 200: 449.
9a. Greenblatt, R. B. 1950. *Med. Clin. North Amer.* 34: 449.
9b. Greenblatt, R. B. 1954. *Obst. & Gynec.* 4: 247.
10. Greenblatt, R. B., and Barfield, W. E. 1952. *Am. J. Obstet. & Gynec.* 63: 153.
11. Greenblatt, R. B., and Jungck, E. C. 1958. *J.A.M.A.* 166 (Mar. 22): 1461.
12. Greenblatt, R. B., and Aydar, C. K. 1961. *Postgrad. Med.* 30L467.
13. Greenblatt, R. B., Hammond, D. O., and Clark, S. L. 1954. 68: 835.
14. Hisaw, F. L. 1935. *Am. J. Obstet. & Gynec.* 29: 638.
15. Jones, G. E. S., and TeLinde, R. W. 1949. *Am. J. Obstet. & Gynec.* 57: 854.
16. McKelvey, J. L., and Samuels, L. T. 1947. *J. Obstet. & Gynec.* 53: 627.
17. Miller, N. F. 1946. *Am. J. Obstet. & Gynec.* 51: 804.
18. Seaman, A. J., and Benson, R. C. 1960. *Am. J. Obstet. & Gynec.* 79: 6.
19. Smith, G. V. S. 1949. *New England J. Med.* 241: 410.
20. Statistics of Dept. of Public Health, Commonwealth of Massachusetts, Boston, Mass.
21. Taymor, M. L., Sturgis, S. H., Goodale, W. T., and Ashbaugh, D. 1960. *Obstet. & Gynec.* 16: 571.
22. Zuckerman, S. 1937. *Proc. Roy. Soc. London*, ser. B, 124: 150.

X

Robert B. Greenblatt, M.D., C.M.
THE MENOPAUSE AND ITS MANAGEMENT

INTRODUCTION

The menopause and its management presents an ever-recurring subject for discussion. In spite of the extensive literature on the subject, opinion is still divided as to the indications for it and what constitutes the most satisfactory approach to treatment. This is understandable and is due as much to the protean nature of the disturbance as it is to individual experience in the management of patients. The problem may best be examined by a consideration of the physiopathology of the menopause and its accompanying symptoms. This should provide the clue for effective management [1], [5].

A better term for "the menopausal syndrome" is "the climacteric." "Menopause" merely means the cessation of menses. The menopause is the period in a woman's life when decline in balanced ovarian function is accompanied by cessation of the menstrual flow. It is another rung in the ladder of a woman's progression through life; it is the climacteric. From the stage of reproductivity she steps into the period of middle-life, free from the responsibility, the stresses, the hazards and trials associated with childbirth. Actually, declining ovarian function is a safeguard against childbirth, but the loss of hormonal support may bring on a train of symptoms which one physician may term psychoneurotic and another physician may term menopausal [10]. This period of a woman's life may be spoken of as a change of life, not merely cessation of menses, not merely an interim which lasts for a few weeks, a few months, a few years. Actually, it is a transition from one way of life to a new one; from one set of environmental influences to a new set, i. e., a new hormonal environment. An analogy may well be drawn from the experience of people who live in the low lands or at sea level and who change their abode by migrating to a high-altitude area. These individuals may find themselves dyspneic. Time is needed in order to become accustomed to the change, not only in environment but also in the culture and manners of the populace about

159

them. One person may adapt rapidly, another slowly, while another fails to make a suitable adjustment. So, too, the woman in the climacteric finds herself in a new altitude, a new hormonal environment, to which it may take weeks, or months, or years to acclimate herself. [4].

The symptomatology and the untoward effects of the climacteric may be divided into three groups: (1) The signs and symptoms resulting from autonomic nervous system imbalance, i.e., hot flashes, cold flashes, sweats, palpitations, spasms, and formication; (2) those deriving from psychogenic disturbances are insomnia, crying spells, depression, apprehension, and nervousness; (3) the symptoms caused by metabolic disorders, including atrophic vulvovaginitis, urinary bladder dysfunction, osteoporosis, myalgias, migranoid headaches, and various catabolic phenomena (Table 10-1). The signs and symptoms may vary from the very mild to the intolerable. Management will then involve measures ranging from simple reassurance to the use of such preparations as will provide relief with minimum hazards.

Table 10-1. Symptoms of the climacteric classified according to causes, i.e., autonomic nervous system imbalance, psychogenic, and metabolic.

Autonomic N. S.	Psychogenic	Metabolic
hot flashes	apprehension	demineralization
formication	depression	myalgia
globus hystericus	insomnia	skin atrophy
perspiration	nervousness	senile vaginitis
spasms	headaches	incontinence
palpitations	frigidity	arthritism

A knowledge of certain physiologic aspects of the problem helps to insure a better understanding of what takes place at this time in a woman's life. Why it is that the woman who has primary ovarian failure, and who has never menstruated, does not experience hot flashes? The syndrome of the climacteric is associated with an estrogen deficiency; nevertheless, the woman with primary ovarian failure does not experience menopausal symptoms in spite of her estrogen lack. The autonomic nervous system ordinarily is tempered and influenced by gonadal hormones from approximately ten years to the age of 50. When this hormonal support is suddenly withdrawn, the patient experiences hot flashes, sweats, and many other symptoms associated with autonomic nervous system imbalance. Actually, if a patient with primary ovarian failure is treated with estrogens for a period of years, so that the autonomic nervous system becomes sensitized by estrogenic therapy, she too will experience hot flashes on withdrawal of the hormonal support.

Another physiologic fact that needs explanation is the occurrence of a high urinary gonadotropin titer in menopausal women. The high

pituitary gonadotropins have been blamed for the symptoms of menopause. Actually, high urinary gonadotropin titers are found in women
with ovarian failure and in eunuchoid males with testicular failure.
These people do not experience symptoms of the menopause. Urinary
gonadotropin titers in a menopausal patient usually are found to be
anywhere from 52 to 208 mouse units per 24 hours. On administering
estrogenic therapy over a period of several weeks, the titer falls to
normal values which are between 6 and 52 mouse units per 24 hours.
Some weeks to months after cessation of therapy there is, in most
women, a gradual return of urinary gonadotropin titers to high levels
(Fig. 10-1). The estrogen deficiency caused by the senescence of the
ovary is the culpable factor in the induction of the menopausal syndrome, not the pituitary secretion.

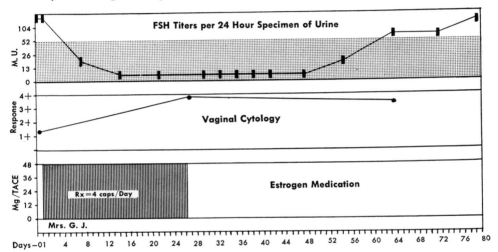

Fig. 10-1. Urinary FSH titers fell while the patient was on estrogen therapy (12 mg
TACE q. i. d.). When, after 26 days, the treatment was discontinued, the vaginal
cytology remained estrogenic but the urinary gonadotrophin titers gradually rose to
pretreatment levels by the 80th day. However, in spite of the rise in FSH titers, the
hot flashes were held in abeyance.

The treatment of the menopause varies among physicians the world
over. There are many who believe that this is a normal physiologic
process and therefore needs no therapy other than assurance. Other
physicians believe that tranquilizers or sedation are sufficient to amel-
iorate the symptoms. Many women need nothing more than encourage-
ment and many may benefit by sedation with phenobarbital, bromides,
or tranquilizers. But the fact remains that we are not treating simply
the psychogenic disturbance, but the metabolic disturbance as well.
Sedation, tranquilizers, and assurance will not prevent the slow onset
of demineralization of bone. The attrition that takes place in the sub-
cutaneous tissue, the atrophy of the vulva, vagina, and many other

tissues in the body, are part of the metabolic changes which are not amenable to therapy with sedation.

Many years ago a prominent gynecologist delivered an address in which he claimed as good results in treatment with a placebo as with hormonal therapy. This statement was challenged, and at the behest of one of the pharmaceutical houses a double blind study was undertaken by Greenblatt's group. Four preparations—a placebo, an estrogen, a combination of estrogen and androgen, and an androgen—were made available [9]. The tablets were labeled and identified only as Nos. 1, 2, 3, and 4. Table 10-2, shows that the patient experienced complete relief with Nos. 1 and 2, but no relief with No. 4. Tables 10-3 and 10-4 afford some idea of the complexity of the problem. For instance, in Table 10-3 the patient obtained relief at first with tablet No. 4, but on continuous therapy with No. 4, the hot flashes returned; complete relief was obtained with No. 1. When the data were finally analyzed, it was correctly concluded that the tablets labeled No. 1 were the estrogen, No. 2 the estrogen-androgen mixture, No. 3 the androgen, and No. 4 the placebo. (The occurrence of uterine bleeding was a clue to the content of No. 1; marked increase in libido with tablet No. 3 offered a clue to its identity. Study of the vaginal cytology was also revealing in these comparative studies, and thus a number of factors entered into play in the analysis of the content of the four preparations.)

Table 10-2.

Mrs. J.S., w.f. 52. Menopause. Hot flashes and formication. (Hysterectomy.)

AE	1	2	3	4	
July	X				Complete relief. Slight increase in libido.
Aug.					Sumptoms returned 3 wks. after stopping AE-1.
Sept.		X			90% relief. Increased libido, nervousness.
Oct.					
Nov.			X		Better than AE-2 or AE-1.
Dec.					Recurrence of symptoms.
Jan.				X	No relief. Smear 2-3 plus.
Feb.		X			80% relief. Occasional hot flashes. Smear 3 plus.
Mar.		X			Not as good as AE-1 now.
Apr.				X	No relief. Complete return of symptoms.

It is of interest to note that 17 per cent of the patients on the placebo tablet obtained relief, whereas about 90 per cent of patients on the estrogen-androgen combination obtained relief (Table 10-5). Thus, there is quite a marked contrast in the effectiveness of placebo therapy and specific therapy. It is also interesting to note that patients preferred tablet No. 2. This estrogen-androgen combination not only decreased the hot flashes but also imparted a greater feeling of well-being [6], [9]. Consequently, over the years, Greenblatt has employed in the treatment of the climacteric not only an estrogen but usually a mild androgen along with it [10].

Table 10-3.

Mrs. H. G. O. , w. f. 44. Menopause. Hot flashes—severe (previously controlled with estrogens but had severe bout of uterine bleeding following estrogen therapy).

AE	1	2	3	4	
June	X				Complete relief. Excessive withdrawal bleeding.
July					
Aug.		X			Complete relief. Almost normal period.
Sept.			X		Recurrence of symptoms, no relief.
Oct.				X	Hot flashes worse than ever before.
Nov.		X			Complete relief. Normal withdrawal period.
Dec.			X		No relief, recurrence of symptoms.
Jan.				X	No relief. Hot flashes severe (20-30 per day).
Feb.	X				Complete relief of symptoms.

Patient preferred AE-2 because withdrawal bleeding was controlled and was much less than with AE-1. Both preparations gave equally good results as far as amelioration of hot flashes was concerned.

Hot flashes experienced during the daytime may be alleviated in a measure by sedation or tranquilizing agents, but the hot flashes which occur during the night and awaken a patient from sleep are not necessarily alleviated by tranquilizers. Table 10-6 illustrates this point. It would appear that the hot flashes escape from the control of the central nervous system while the patient is asleep. The same patient, when given estrogen alone or estrogen-androgen combination, obtained excellent relief of the hot flashes during the day time and during the night as well. There is, therefore, no real substitute for specific therapy.

There are many aspects of the climacteric which are neglected because of failure to understand that this is a period of life which is not confined to the few months or the year or two immediately after the cessation of menses [3]. Many years later a patient may experience senile vaginitis, with discharge and pruritus, and all the discomfort that attends it. Such patients respond much more readily to specific therapy than to nonspecific therapy with douches and creams. The administration of estrogens, in the form of suppositories inserted into the vaginal canal, or the oral or parenteral administration of estrogens,

Table 10-4.

Mrs. L.C.M., w.f. 39. Menopause. Hot flashes and nervousness.
Smear 2 plus. (Hysterectomy.)

AE	1	2	3	4	
June	X				Satisfactory relief of symptoms. Nervous.
July		X			Better than AE-1, less nervous. Smear 3-4 plus.
Aug.			X		Better than AE-1 or AE-2.
Sept.				X	Very well; no change.
Oct.				X	Very well; no change.
Nov.				X	Not so well. Backache. Smear 3 plus.
Dec.				X	Complete return of symptoms.
Jan.				X	Worse than ever. Smear 2 plus.
Feb.				X	Nervous. Severe hot flashes. Smear 2 plus.
Mar.	X				Relief of all symptoms. Calm. Smear 4 plus.

Patient at first obtained satisfactory results with AE-1, 2, 3 and 4, administered in that order, but symptoms recurred on continued therapy with AE-4 and were entirely relieved by AE-1.

Table 10-5. Analysis of response to therapy with AE preparations in 74 private patients and 28 clinic patients with 284 courses of therapy.

Therapy	Courses of therapy		Percentage of patients				
	Private	Clinic	With nausea	With increased libido	With acne, hoarseness, or hirsutism	With intact uterus and bleeding following treatment	With no improvement
AE-1 Diethylstilbestrol, 0.25 mg.	67	21	30.5	12.3	0	34.2	3.1
AE-2 Diethylstilbestrol, 0.25 mg. Methyltestosterone, 5.0 mg.	54	19	4.0	23.5	13.2	30.5	10.4
AE-3 Methyltestosterone, 5.0 mg.	44	19	5.2	42.0	12.8	0.98	23.6
AE-4 Placebo	36	24	3.6	1.8	0	0	83.8

Table 10-6. Hot flashes occurring during the daytime may at times be alleviated by sedation or autonomic depressant drugs. However, in this case, the flashes which occurred during the night escaped from the influence of such treatment. When an estrogen-androgen preparation was added to Bellergal, the hot flashes, both day and night, were brought under control.

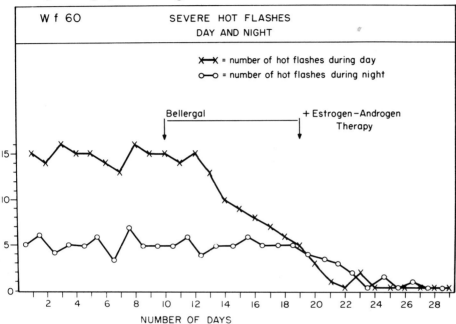

may bring about rapid relief of the discomfort and symptoms. Figure 10-2a represents a histologic section showing the atrophy of the vaginal mucosa in patients with senile vaginitis. Note that the cells comprising the mucosa, i.e., the cells lining the vagina, are only two to five layers in thickness. Under normal circumstances the vaginal mucosa is lined by 25 to 30 layers of cells (Fig. 10-2b). The atrophic condition of the vagina can readily be restored to its full thickness by estrogen therapy, accompanied by the cessation of symptoms.

Another condition seen in patients with an estrogen deficiency, particularly in the late climacteric, is kraurosis vulvae. Kraurosis vulvae is a symptoms-complex and it is not due to estrogen deficiency alone. Figure 10-3a is a typical example of kraurosis vulvae. Note the thick, blanched skin and the atrophy of the vulva. In Fig. 10-3b, the thickening of the keratin layer, the atrophy of the epithelial cell layer, and the infiltration of the subepithelial layer by a myxomatous type of material are demonstrated by the histologic section. That kraurosis vulvae is due to more than an estrogen deficiency is suggested by studies which Greenblatt previously reported on 25 patients, 24

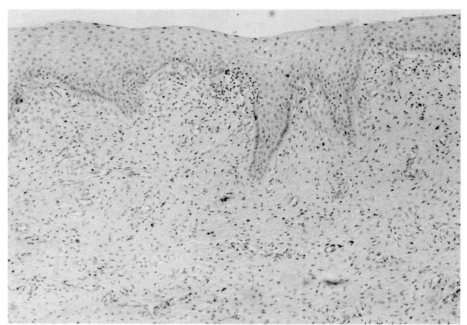

Fig. 10-2a.   Photomicrograph of histologic section of biopsy of vaginal mucosa in estrogen deficiency states.

of whom were found to have an absence of free hydrochloric acid in the gastric secretions [7].   By way of treatment, the addition of hydrochloric acid orally to the oral or parenteral use of estrogens, and the local application to the vulva of a cream containing estrogen and hydrocortisone, have offered the best results in our experience.   This therapy assuages the discomfort and intense itching and thus minimizes the desire for scratching with resultant traumatization of the labia.   It is my own belief that it is the trauma which predisposes to development of leucoplakia and cancer.   If pruritus can be reduced to a minimum, obviating the need for scratching, carcinoma of the vulva, in all probability, may not arise, and such a patient may be treated by conservative measures for the rest of her life [7].   Although cure may not be obtained, partial or complete alleviation of the discomfort may be expected.   Surgery is not the answer to the problem, although surgical excision of the vulvae is frequently advocated.   The kraurotic areas frequently persist around the point of excision and in the perianal region, and the unfortunate patient continues to suffer the full extent of the symptoms.

The osteoporosis that develops in the postmenopausal period is also a part of the climacteric [1], [2], [12].   A certain number of patients will develop marked demineralization of bone with compression

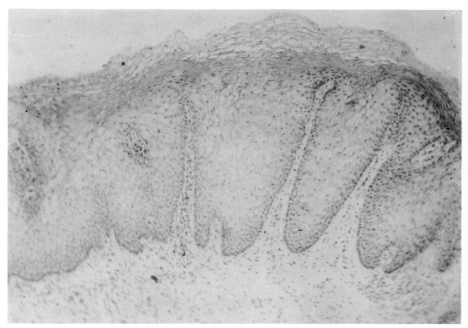

Fig. 10-2b. Photomicrograph of histologic section of biopsy of vaginal mucosa under normal estrogen stimulation.

fractures of the vertebrae. Fractures of the ribs, and more often fracture of the head of the femur, may result from the slightest trauma. Estrogens stimulate osteoblastic cells to lay down calcium, and if the proper matrix is present the loss of calcium from bones is minimal. It is true that marked demineralization does not take place in all post-menopausal women. Unknown factors are involved. Nonetheless, the continuous administration of an estrogen to keep the osteoblasts active, and of an androgen to stimulate the protein matrix to hold the calcium, may prevent the onset of marked demineralization with the sequellae of invalidism due to collapsed vertebrae. Figure 10-4 shows X-ray studies on a patient whose ovaries were removed sometime in her thirties. Substitutional therapy was not given her. Twenty-five years later she presented the complaint of severe backache caused by marked osteoporosis with collapsed vertebrae. With the administration of estrogens and androgens, further collapse of the vertebrae did not occur. Although remineralization was not evident in subsequent X rays, there was marked clinical improvement with remarkable alleviation of back pain. It would be judicious to have X-ray studies done on all menopausal and postmenopausal patients. If evidence of demineralization is present, one can prescribe a monthly injection of a long-acting estrogen-androgen preparation, or oral therapy with an estrogen alone or with small doses of

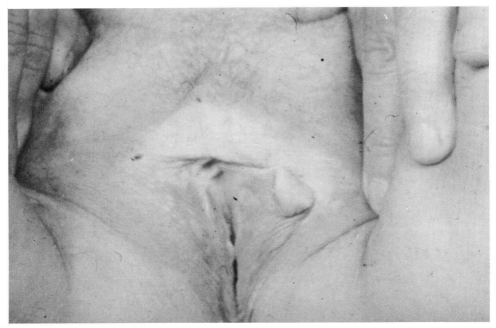

Fig. 10-3a. Kraurosis vulvae. Note blanching and thickening of skin and atrophy of labia.

an androgen for three weeks in each month, in the hope of preventing further demineralization of bone.

Mention should be made of the arthralgias which seem to blossom in the postmenopausal period. Many women complain of the beginning or worsening of arthritic changes and osteoarthritis at this time. Figure 10-5 illustrates a patient who was a typist. Flexible fingers were a necessity in her employment. Along with other symptoms of the menopause, she had experienced a worsening of the arthritic condition. X rays of the hands showed marked osteoarthritis of the interphalangeal joints. She was given estrogen-androgen medication, and as long as she continued on this therapy she was able to work and use her hands satisfactorily. Hormonal therapy is not a cure for osteoarthritis and many patients may not respond to it, but when a woman develops this condition during the postmenopausal period, it is worthwhile to administer estrogens and androgens rather than corticoids. It should be warned that corticoids given in the postmenopausal period will hasten the development of further osteoporosis, and are a threat to the body's mineral economy [11]. Where equally good results can be obtained, the use of safer preparations such as estrogens and androgens is preferable.

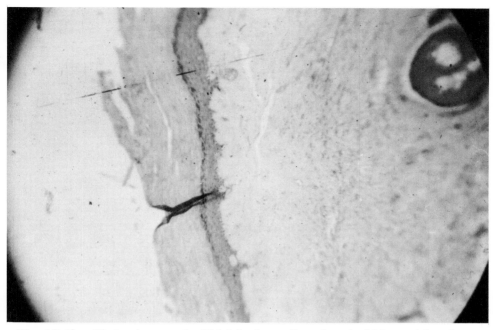

Fig. 10-3b. Photomicrograph of histologic section of vaginal biopsy taken from patient in Fig. 10-3a. Note the thick keratin layer, the atrophy of the epidermis, and the myxomatous type of degeneration of the subepithelial layers.

Urinary frequency, nocturia, or stress incontinence are frequently present without an anatomic or pathologic basis, but as concomitants of the menopause which may be ameliorated by estrogens or preferably androgens [8]. Though moderate doses of estrogens help in arresting this complaint, it should be recalled that administration of massive doses of estrogen to postmenopausal women with breast carcinoma may bring on urinary frequency. This does not occur when such patients are treated with massive doses of androgens. Moreover, in the management of urinary frequency and nocturia, androgens yield as good or better results than those obtained with moderate estrogen dosage.

Menopausal headache is one of the complaints that frequently proves recalcitrant to simple estrogen therapy, although estrogens as a rule are satisfactory in arresting flushes, formication, sweats, nervousness, etc. However, administration of androgens, alone and in some instances along with estrogens, have afforded relief from severe incapacitating headaches that have been mistaken for migraine.

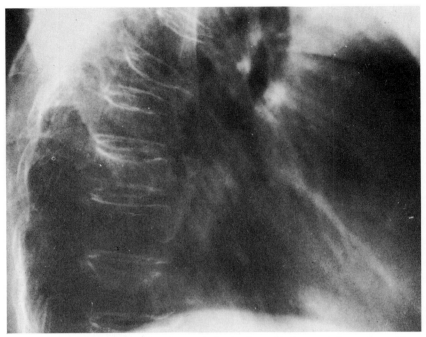

Fig. 10-4. Severe demineralization of the bodies of the vertebrae in a 60-year-old patient in whom the ovaries were removed 25 years earlier.

CONCLUSION

The menopausal syndrome, or the syndrome of the climacteric, occupies a woman's life from the time the ovaries begin to decline to the end of life. The climacteric is not confined to a brief period of several months or a few years. While it is true that the menopause is a physiological process and represents a period of adjustment to a new hormonal internal milieu, withholding measures that may make the transition smoother or prevent disabling pathological processes—be they psychological, neurological, or metabolic—when they are clearly amenable to treatment, is unrealistic. Many women may be restored from a chronic state of semi-invalidism to mental and physical health with the judicious use of therapy with steroid hormones. There is no justifiable reason to withhold hormone therapy from the patient in the climacteric when its use can make life more pleasant and prevent some of the crippling, incapacitating, and uncomfortable complications of this period.

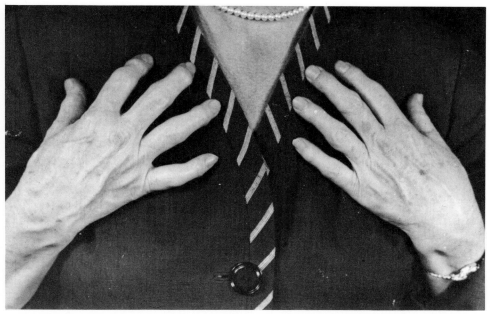

Fig. 10-5. Aggravation of osteoarthritis during the menopause. This patient responded well to estrogen-androgen medication.

REFERENCES

1. Albright, F. 1947. *Ann. Int. Med.* 27: 861.
2. Albright, F. 1947. *Recent Progr. Hormone Res.* 1: 293.
3. Allen, W. M. 1951. *Proc. Second Sympos. on Clinical Problems of Advancing Years*, 27.
4. Brown, M. L., Lucente, E. R., Alesbury, J. M., and Perloff, W. H. 1951. *Am. J. Obstet. & Gynec.* 61: 200.
5. Collett, M. E. 1949. *J. Appl. Physiol.* 1: 629.
6. Glass, S. J. 1950. *J. Clin. Endocrinol.* 10: 1616.
7. Greenblatt, R. B. 1950. *Postgrad. Med.* 8: 471.
8. Greenblatt, R. B. 1952. *Geriatrics* 7: 263.
9. Greenblatt, R. B., Barfield, W. E., Garner, J. F., Calk, G. L., and Harrod, J. P. 1950. *J. Clin. Endocrinol.* 10: 1547.
10. Greenblatt, R. B., Barfield, W. E., and Jungck, E. C. 1962. *Canadian M. A. J.* 86: 113.
11. Moreno Martinez, O., and Greenblatt, R. B. 1960. *Geriatrics* 15: 555.
12. Reifenstein, E. C., Jr., and Albright, F. 1947. *J. Clin. Invest.* 26: 24.

XI

J. A. Loraine, D.Sc., F.R.C.P.E., E. T. Bell, B.Sc.,
and H. Schmidt-Elmendorff, M.D.

BIOLOGICAL PROPERTIES OF GONADOTROPIC HORMONES

The work described in this chapter has been reported in detail elsewhere [16], [17], [19]; the present communication is mainly concerned with the conclusions reached in investigations in the following areas:

1. The biological activity of various gonadotropin preparations.
2. The effect of 6M urea on gonadotropic activity.
3. Gonadotropic activity in the body fluids of pregnant mares.

THE BIOLOGICAL ACTIVITY OF VARIOUS GONADOTROPIN PREPARATIONS

Hormones Tested

These were as follows:

1. Follicle-stimulating hormone (ovine-NIH-FSH-S1).
2. Luteinizing hormone (ovine-NIH-LH-S1).
3. Follicle-stimulating hormone (human - C. E. R. U. preparation). This was prepared in Edinburgh by the method of Li, et al. [10].
4. Human Menopausal Gonadotropin—HMG-20A. [4]
5. International Reference Preparation for Human Menopausal Gonadotropin (I. R. P.) This preparation has been shown to be approximately equipotent with HMG-20A [4].
6. Human Menopausal Gonadotropin—Pergonal. This material has been shown to have a higher specific activity than the I. R. P. Its biological properties are described elsewhere [15], [17].
7. Pregnant mare's serum gonadotropin (PMSG)—international standard.
8. Human Chorionic Gonadotropin (HCG)—international standard.

Bioassay Methods

These were six in number and were performed according to the specifications of the authors listed below.

1. Ovarian weight test in intact immature mice treated with large dosages of HCG—*augmentation test* [3].

2. Ovarian ascorbic acid depletion test in intact immature rats pretreated with PMSG and HCG—*O. A. A. D. test* [14].

3. Ventral prostatic weight test in hypophysectomized immature male rats—*hypophysectomized rat prostate* (H. R. P.) *test* [11].

4. Uterine weight test in intact immature mice [11].

5. Uterine weight test in intact immature rats [5].

6. Ovarian weight test in intact immature mice [9].

Method 1 measures predominantly FSH [20], while Methods 2 and 3 are highly specific indicators of LH activity [12], [14], [16]. Methods 4, 5, and 6 are nonspecific tests measuring a mixture of FSH and LH activities and provide an estimate of what may conveniently be referred to as "total gonadotropic activity." In the great majority of assays performed, the I. R. P. was used as the reference preparation and the unknown material assayed in terms of this substance.

Results

These are shown in Tables 11-1 to 11-6. Practically all the assays were of a symmetrical four-point design in which two dose levels of the reference preparation were compared with two dose levels of the unknown preparation. In the Tables, "N" represents the number of animals used in each assay. The indices of precision (λ), relative potencies and fiducial limits of error were calculated by the method of Gaddum [8].

Table 11-1. Biological Activity of NIH-FSH in Terms of I. R. P. Using Various Assay Methods*

Bioassay	Design	N	λ	R. P.	Fiducial limits (P = 0.95)	Mean R. P.
Augmentation test	2+2	12	0.28	61.1	27.5-177.0	68.1
	2+2	14	0.35	105.4	54.1-244.6	
	2+2	14	0.17	67.0	40.2-114.6	
	2+2	16	0.26	39.0	14.4-80.3	
O. A. A. D. test	2+2	20	0.45	28.2	19.4-94.9	28.7
	2+2	20	0.19	40.7	29.7-59.8	
	2+2	20	0.38	17.2	8.9-33.4	
Mouse uterus test	2+2	15	0.13	14.5	6.1-28.5	15.4
	2+2	15	0.10	16.3	10.8-23.2	

*Schmidt-Elmendorff, et. al. [17]

1. *NIH-FSH* (Table 11-1). The mean FSH activity of this material is approximately 68 times and its LH activity 30 times that of the I. R. P. The relative potency as estimated by the mouse uterus test was found to be considerably lower than that obtained by the other two methods.

2. *NIH-LH* (Table 11-2). This material is a highly purified LH preparation being approximately 2,000 times more active than the I. R. P.

Table 11-2. LH Activity of NIH-LH in Terms of I. R. P.
- O. A. A. D. Test*

Design	N	λ	R. P.	Fiducial limits (P = 0.95)	Mean R. P.
2+2	20	0.29	2670	1362–4779	
2+2	20	0.36	3190	2200–4562	
2+2	20	0.19	1361	1007–1946	2051
2+2	20	0.26	1811	1014–2789	
2+2	20	0.22	1221	867–1721	

*Schmidt-Elmendorff, et al. [17]

3. *Human Pituitary FSH* (Table 11-3). This material is very rich in FSH activity, being 96 times more active than the I. R. P. Its LH activity was much lower than that of the NIH-LH using the O. A. A. D. test but was 12 times higher than that of the I. R. P. using the H. R. P. test. The gonadotropic potency of this preparation as estimated by the mouse uterus test, in terms of the I. R. P., lay between its FSH and LH activities.

Table 11-3. Biological Activity of Human Pituitary FSH in Terms of Various Reference Materials*

Reference material	Bioassay	Design	N	λ	R. P.	Fiducial limits (P = 0.95)	Mean R. P.
NIH–FSH	Augmentation test	2+2	16	0.28	1.27	0.41–3.26	
		2+2	16	0.20	1.04	0.80–1.30	1.38
		2+2	16	0.30	1.83	0.15–3.95	
NIH–LH	O. A. A. D. test	2+2	20	0.29	0.016	0.007–0.027	
		2+2	20	0.27	0.066	0.044–0.101	0.054
		2+2	20	0.19	0.081	0.079–0.083	
		2+2	20	0.17	0.052	0.038–0.071	
I. R. P.	Augmentation test	2+2	16	0.23	79.4	39.7–159.6	
		2+2	16	0.19	93.0	50.4–222.9	96.3
		2+2	16	0.24	116.5	31.4–215.5	
	H. R. P. test	2+2	12	0.12	12.0	6.3–18.4	12.0
	Mouse uterus test	2+2	16	0.10	66.0	50.2–85.1	69.0
		2+2	16	0.12	72.0	51.5–98.8	

*Schmidt-Emendorff, et al. [17]

4. *Pergonal* (Table 11-4). This preparation has ten times more FSH and five times more LH activity than the I. R. P. Estimates of its LH activity obtained by the O. A. A. D. and H. R. P. tests agreed well as did estimates of its gonadotropic potency by the mouse uterus and rat uterus tests.

Table 11-4. Biological Activity of Pergonal in Terms of I. R. P. Using Various Assay Methods*

Bioassay	Design	N	λ	R. P.	Fiducial limits (P = 0.95)	Mean R. P.
Augmentation	2+2	16	0.20	10.5	5.7-17.3	
	2+2	16	0.18	9.1	5.1-14.4	10.05
	2+2	14	0.32	10.5	5.8-33.1	
O. A. A. D. test	2+2	20	0.47	3.60	1.60-11.10	
	2+2	20	0.27	10.90	6.20-25.50	
	2+2	20	0.18	3.50	2.50-5.40	
	2+2	20	0.20	3.53	2.65-4.87	5.3
	2+2	20	0.27	6.08	4.07-10.21	
	2+2	20	0.33	4.10	2.50-7.30	
H. R. P. test	2+1	12	0.16	5.0	2.3-6.6	5.0
Mouse uterus test	2+2	16	0.09	11.9	9.1-14.9	
	2+2	16	0.12	12.2	8.3-16.4	12.0
Rat uterus test	2+2	12	0.17	11.0	4.3-21.7	
	2+1	9	0.13	12.0	7.1-16.7	11.5

*Schmidt-Elmendorff, et al. [17]

5. *PMSG* (Table 11-5). This material has more FSH and less LH activity than the I. R. P. The gonadotropic potency of PMSG as estimated by the mouse uterus test was higher than either its FSH or LH activities. The potency ratio obtained by the mouse uterus test was approximately double that obtained by the mouse ovarian weight test.

6. *HCG* (Table 11-6). The LH activity of HCG in terms of the I. R. P. and Pergonal is shown in Table 11-6. It will be noted that its activity was only 1.71 times that of the I. R. P. and less than half that of Pergonal. When HCG was assayed by the mouse uterus test in terms of the I. R. P., significant deviation from parallelism occurred (P < 0.001), and the assay was therefore invalid.

Summary

1. NIH-LH is a preparation of high specific activity, being approximately 2,000 times more potent than the I. R. P.

2. Human Pituitary FSH contains the highest FSH activity of any preparation tested.

Table 11-5. Biological Activity of PMSG in Terms of I. R. P. Using Various Assay Methods*

Bioassay	Design	N	λ	R. P.	Fiducial limits (P = 0.95)	Mean R. P.
Augmentation test	2+2	12	0.18	1.6	0.9-3.2	1.3
	2+2	14	0.08	1.3	1.0-1.6	
	2+2	14	0.25	0.85	0.3-2.1	
O. A. A. D. test	2+2	20	0.21	0.58	0.42-0.79	
	2+2	20	0.23	0.52	0.36-0.75	
	2+2	20	0.27	0.66	0.43-1.02	0.62
	2+2	20	0.41	0.98	0.52-2.40	
	2+2	20	0.40	0.36	0.12-0.71	
Mouse uterus test	2+2	16	0.08	2.6	2.0-3.2	
	2+2	16	0.11	3.1	2.3-4.2	2.9
Mouse ovarian weight test	2+2	16	0.10	1.5	1.2-2.0	
	2+2	16	0.10	1.3	1.0-1.7	1.4

Reference material HMG-20A.

*Schmidt-Elmendorff, et al. [17]

Table 11-6. LH Activity of HCG in Terms of I. R. P. and Pergonal - O. A. A. D. Test*

Reference material	Design	N	λ	R. P.	Fiducial limits (P - 0.95)	Mean R. P.
I. R. P.	2+2	20	0.27	1.27	0.84-1.96	
	2+2	20	0.21	1.78	1.38-2.58	
	2+2	20	0.31	2.50	1.55-4.75	1.71
	2+2	20	0.35	1.27	0.75-2.30	
Pergonal	2+2	20	0.18	0.53	0.41-0.70	
	2+2	20	0.28	0.42	0.27-0.65	0.43
	2+2	20	0.24	0.33	0.23-0.47	

*Schmidt-Elmendorff, et al. [17]

3. Pergonal contains ten times more FSH and five times more LH activity than the I. R. P. It appears to have lost half of its LH activity during preparation.

4. PMSG contains, in addition to its FSH activity, a considerable amount of LH activity; the ratio FSH/LH was approximately 2:1.

5. The International Standard for HCG is a relatively weak LH preparation being only twice as active as the I. R. P.

6. Results obtained by the mouse uterus test do not bear any constant relationship to those obtained by either FSH or LH specific methods.

THE EFFECT OF 6M UREA ON GONADOTROPIC ACTIVITY

Ellis [6], [7] has shown that when pituitary gonadotropin extracts are incubated with 6M urea, LH activity is greatly reduced while FSH activity is virtually unaffected. The present study was designed to extend Ellis' observations and to investigate the effect of 6M urea on the LH, FSH, and total gonadotropic activity of preparations from a number of different sources.

Design of Investigation

The hormones tested were (1) NIH-FSH, (2) NIH-LH, (3) Pergonal, (4) PMSG, and (5) HCG (see page 172). The bioassay methods used were (1) the *O. A. A. D. test*, (2) the *augmentation test*, and (3) the *mouse uterus test* (see page 173). The hormones were incubated at $40° \pm 1°$C for 24 hours using both 6M urea and distilled water. Assays were conducted using both a four-point and a three-point design, and the results were calculated by the method of Gaddum [8].

1. *O. A. A. D. Method.*

In Table 11-7 is shown the remaining LH activity when the hormones were incubated with 6M urea. It will be noted that NIH-LH and NIH-FSH either in combination or alone lost more than 94 per cent of their original LH activity. In the case of Pergonal and HCG a comparable amount of LH activity was destroyed, but with PMSG a mean of 46 per cent of the activity remained.

In the incubations with distilled water involving NIH-LH, NIH-FSH, HCG, and PMSG the losses of LH activity were very small and in all experiments the fiducial limits of error (P = 0.95) included the figure of 100 per cent. In the case of Pergonal more than 50 per cent of the activity was destroyed by this form of treatment and this suggests that the LH activity of Pergonal is less stable than that of the other gonadotropins studied.

2. *Augmentation Test.*

In Table 11-8 is shown the remaining FSH activity when NIH-FSH and Pergonal were incubated with 6M urea. It is apparent that in the case of NIH-FSH very little activity was lost, the mean figure for the residual activity being 91 per cent. With Pergonal 93 per cent of the FSH activity was destroyed.

3. *Mouse Uterus Test.*

In Table 11-9 is shown the residual total gonadotropic activity when the hormones were incubated with 6M urea. It will be noted that the degree of inactivation was greater with NIH-FSH than with PMSG;

Table 11-7. Residual LH Activity Following Incubation with 6M Urea
- O. A. A. D. Method*

Materials tested	Design	λ	Residual activity (%)	Fiducial limits (%) (P = 0.95)	Mean residual activity (%)
NIH-LH	2+2	0.29	4.4	2.1-8.7	5.7
"	2+1	0.12	7.1	5.8-8.6	
NIH-FSH	2+2	0.34	0.2	0.04-0.9	4.1
"	2+1	0.16	8.0	7.0-9.0	
NIH-FSH + NIH-LH	2+1	0.45	1.8	0.2-13.2	1.8
HCG	2+1	0.12	6.8	5.3-8.7	3.6
"	2+2	0.14	0.5	0.4-0.5	
PMSG	2+1	0.13	56.0	42.5-73.4	46.2
"	2+2	0.15	36.4	26.2-49.5	
Pergonal	2+1	0.45	10.5	4.2-28.3	6.4
"	2+1	0.33	2.4	1.6-3.4	

*Schmidt-Elmendorff, et al. [18]

however, with Pergonal more than 90 per cent of the activity was lost.
In the control incubations with distilled water neither NIH-FSH nor
PMSG lost appreciable activity. In the two experiments involving
Pergonal the residual activities were respectively 49 per cent and 91
per cent.

Table 11-8. Residual FSH Activity Following Incubation with 6M Urea
- Augmentation Test*

Materials tested	Design	λ	Residual activity (%)	Fiducial limits (%) (P = 0.95)	Mean residual activity (%)
NIH-FSH	2+1	0.14	117	81-254	91
"	2+1	0.17	65	35-142	
Pergonal	2+1	0.17	7	2-11	7
"	2+1	0.18	6	3-10	

*Schmidt-Elmendorff, et al. [18]

Table 11-9. Residual "Total Gonadotropic" Activity Following Incubation
with 6M Urea - Mouse Uterus Test*

Materials tested	Design	λ	Residual activity (%)	Fiducial limits (%) (P = 0.95)	Mean residual activity (%)
NIH–FSH	2+2	0.10	28	20–40	
"	2+2	0.09	54	44–68	
"	2+2	0.11	52	46–72	50
"	2+1	0.13	43	30–70	
"	2+1	0.12	74	51–152	
PMSG	2+1	0.12	37	26–77	67
"	2+1	0.10	97	65–198	
Pergonal	2+1	0.12	9	7–11	
"	2+1	0.10	7	5–9	8
"	2+1	0.12	7	5–9	

*Schmidt-Elmendorff, et al. [18]

Summary

1. Following incubation with 6M urea, the LH activities of NIH-LH, NIH-FSH, HCG, and Pergonal were almost completely destroyed, while the LH activity of PMSG was reduced to a smaller extent.

2. The FSH activity of NIH-FSH was little affected by incubation with 6M urea.

3. The total gonadotropic activity of NIH-FSH, PMSG, and Pergonal was reduced after incubation with 6M urea, the degree of inactivation being greatest in the case of Pergonal.

4. After control incubations with water, no appreciable loss of biological activity was observed with any hormone other than Pergonal.

GONADOTROPIC ACTIVITY IN THE BODY FLUIDS OF PREGNANT MARES

The purpose of this section is to report the presence of gonadotropic activity in the urine as well as in the serum of the pregnant mare. This finding was noted during an investigation undertaken to determine the action of derivatives of dithiocarbamoylhydrazine (Compounds 22,365 and 33,828, Imperial Chemical Industries Ltd.) on gonadotropic activity in the body fluids of these animals. These compounds have been shown to act as selective inhibitors of pituitary gonadotropic function in rats, dogs, monkeys, and human subjects (Paget, et al. [13]; Bell, et al. [2]). In contradistinction to many pituitary inhibitors previously described, neither compound is a steroid.

Design of Investigation

Three animals were studied, and the results obtained in one of them (Mare 63) are shown in Fig. 11-1. Unextracted serum was employed in all assays; urine samples were precipitated with acetone and washed with ether, and the precipitate was subsequently dissolved in 0.9 per cent saline. This procedure eliminated any possibility of contamination of the final extract by the estrogens which are known to be present in large quantities in the urine of pregnant mares [1].

Bioassay Methods

All assays in serum were performed using the test depending on the enlargement of the ovaries in intact immature mice. In urine samples with a relatively high gonadotropic activity, the same method was used, but in low-titer urines the endpoint of the bioassay was the test depending on uterine enlargement in intact immature mice. Both assays were conducted according to the specifications of Hamburger and Pedersen-Bjergaard [9], and all the results were expressed in terms of the international standard for PMSG. The results of serum assays were expressed as i. u. per liter; in the case of urine samples it was not possible to collect complete 24-hour specimens, and it was therefore necessary to express the results as concentrations (i. u. per liter) rather than as 24-hour excretion values. Approximately 50 per cent of the assays in serum were of a four-point design. The remainder of the assays in serum and all the assays in urine were calculated on a three-point basis.

Results

The data obtained in one of the three animals studied are shown in Figure 11-1.

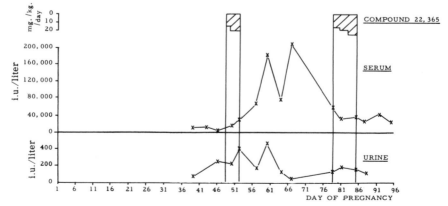

Fig. 11-1. Serum and urinary gonadotropin levels in Mare 63. From Schmidt-Elmendorff, H., Loraine, J.A., Bell, E.T., and Walley, J.K. [19].

It will be noted that high serum gonadotropin values were found from the 50th to the 70th day of pregnancy; thereafter, low readings were encountered. Gonadotropic activity was detected in the urine of this animal from the 7th to the 13th week of gestation; the highest concentration in urine coincided with one of the highest levels in serum, but the mean urinary concentration was approximately 600 times lower than the mean serum level. Compound 22,365 was administered twice during the early stages of pregnancy, but on neither occasion was there any definite effect on serum gonadotropin levels.

The results in the other two animals were similar to those shown in Fig. 11-1. From the evidence reported herein and from the fact that derivatives of dithiocarbamoylhydrazine do not appear to affect HCG excretion in pregnant women (Brown, Fotherby & Loraine—unpublished) it appears reasonable to conclude that they inhibit pituitary rather than placental gonadotropic function.

Summary

1. Gonadotropic activity was detected in the urine as well as in the serum of three pregnant mares. In all cases the readings in urine were much lower than the serum values, but in two animals the pattern of excretion of gonadotropin in urine appeared to follow the serum concentration during the period of investigation.

2. Derivatives of dithiocarbamoylhydrazine had no appreciable effect on gonadotropin levels in either serum or urine and do not appear to influence placental gonadotropic function.

REFERENCES

1. Amoroso, E. C. 1955. *Brit. Med. Bull.* 11: 117.
2. Bell, E. T., Brown, J. B., Fotherby, K., Loraine, J. A., and Robson, J. S. 1962. *J. Endocrinol.* 25: 221.
3. Brown, P. S. 1955. *J. Endocrinol.* 13: 59.
4. Bull. World Health Org. 1960. 22: 563.
5. Diczfalusy, E., and Loraine, J. A. 1955. *J. Clin. Endocrinol.* 15: 424.
6. Ellis, S. 1961a. *Endocrinology* 68: 334.
7. Ellis, S. 1961b. In *Human Pituitary Gonadotropins.* A Workshop Conference, ed. A. Albert, C. C Thomas, Springfield, Ill., 378.
8. Gaddum, J. H. 1953. *Pharm. Rev.* 5: 87.
9. Hamburger, C., and Pedersen-Bjergaard, K. 1937. *Quart. J. Pharm.* 10: 662.
10. Li, C. H., Simpson, Miriam E., and Evans, H. M. 1949. *Science* 109: 445.
11. Loraine, J. A., and Brown, J. B. 1954. *Acta Endocrinol. Copenhagen* 17: 250.

12. Loraine, J. A., and Diczfalusy, E. 1958. *J. Endocrinol.* 17: 425.
13. Paget, G. E., Walpole, A. L. and Richardson, D. N. 1961. *Nature,* London, 192: 1191.
14. Parlow, A. 1961. In *Human Pituitary Gonadotropins.* A Workshop Conference, ed. A. Albert, C. C Thomas, Springfield, Ill., 300.
15. Rosemberg, Eugenia, and Engel, I. 1961. *J. Clin. Endocrinol.* 21: 603.
16. Schmidt-Elmendorff, H., and Loraine, J. A. 1962. *J. Endocrinol.* 23: 413.
17. Schmidt-Elmendorff, H., Loraine, J. A., and Bell, E. T. 1962a. *J. Endocrinol.* 24: 349.
18. Schmidt-Elmendorff, H., Loraine, J. A., and Bell, E. T. 1962b. *J. Endocrinol.* 24: 153.
19. Schmidt-Elmendorff, H., Loraine, J. A., Bell, E. T., and Walley, J. K. 1962c. *J. Endocrinol.* 25: 107.
20. Simpson, Miriam, E. 1961. In *Human Pituitary Gonadotropins.* A Workshop Conference, ed. A. Albert, C. C Thomas, Springfield, Ill., 394.

XII

John A. Loraine, D.Sc., F.R.C.P.E.
SOME CLINICAL APPLICATIONS OF ASSAYS OF PITUITARY GONADOTROPINS IN HUMAN URINE

INTRODUCTION

This chapter deals with three main topics:

1. The excretion of human pituitary gonadotropins (HPG) in normal subjects.

2. HPG excretion in pathological conditions.

3. The effect of various compounds on HPG excretion.

The literature on these subjects up to 1958 has been reviewed previously [16] and the present communication deals mainly with information which has accumulated since that date. Much of the data presented has been obtained in studies conducted by Loraine, et al. in Edinburgh. In these studies the method used for the quantitative determination of HPG in urine was that of Loraine and Brown [22]. In this procedure the urine is extracted by the kaolin-acetone method, the endpoint of the bioassay is the mouse uterus test and results are expressed in terms of the International Reference Preparation for Human Menopausal Gonadotropin (HMG) as "HMG units per 24-hour urine sample."

HPG EXCRETION IN NORMAL SUBJECTS

Children

Most investigators agree that the gonadotropic activity in the urine of children and adolescents is low. Nathanson, et al. [31] were unable to detect HPG in boys before the age of 13 but obtained positive results in girls at the age of 11. Catchpole, et al. [10], who studied HPG output in young and adolescent boys, also found low values and concluded that the titer was related to developmental stature rather than to chronological age.

In a more recent study, P. S. Brown [9] estimated the Follicle-Stimulating Hormone (FSH) and total gonadotropic activity in the urine of boys and girls; the bioassay methods used were the mouse ovarian "augmentation" and mouse uterus tests respectively. He found that both forms of activity were higher in girls than in boys. The figures quoted in prepuberal girls were much higher than any previously reported in the literature, but the reason for this finding is at present obscure.

Normal Men

It has been known for many years that male urine contains HPG activity. In a recent investigation in Edinburgh [24], 40 assays were performed in 28 normal male subjects ranging in age from 20 to 60. The mean HPG excretion was 11.0 HMG units/24 hours and the range (P = 0.95) was from 5.0 to 23.0 HMG units/24 hours.

Normally Menstruating Women

The pattern of excretion of HPG throughout the normal menstrual cycle is now well established. Readings are usually low in the follicular and luteal phases and a peak of excretion is frequently noted at or about the time of ovulation. In 157 assays made in 15 women aged 18 to 57, the mean HPG excretion was 10.0 HMG units/24 hours and the range (P = 0.95) was from 5.0 to 34.0 HMG units/24 hours 24 . In the follicular and luteal phases readings were generally below 15 HMG units/24 hours. At midcycle a gonadotropin peak was observed in approximately 50 per cent of the subjects studied; when this peak occurred, readings as high as 40.0 HMG units/24 hours were obtained.

The relationship between the estrogen and HPG peaks at midcycle in normally menstruating women has been discussed by J. B. Brown, et al. [8]. These workers found that in none of nine subjects studied did the HPG peak precede the estrogen peak. In some women the two peaks coincided, while in others the HPG peak postdated the estrogen peak by periods as long as 72 hours.

The reason for this finding, which cannot be reconciled with the currently accepted hypotheses on the hormonal control of the menstrual cycle, is at present obscure. One possibility might be that the low renal clearance of HPG is responsible and that, if it were practicable to conduct HPG assays in plasma as well as in urine throughout the cycle, the peak concentration in blood might be found to occur earlier than that in urine. An alternative explanation is that, in the initiation and maintenance of the menstrual rhythm in humans, the ovary is more autonomous than has previously been supposed, and that changes in gonadotropin secretion are the result rather than the cause of alterations in the production of ovarian hormones. That this concept of "ovarian autonomy" is not as improbable as it may at first appear is indicated by the observations of J. B. Brown, et al. [6], [7] and Bell, et al. [4] who showed that the progestational compound 17α-ethynyl-17β-hydroxy-19-norandrost-4-en-3-one (norethisterone) and the dithiocarbamoylhydrazine derivative, Compound 33,828, are capable of inhibiting ovulation, as judged by estrogen and pregnanediol excretion, without affecting urinary HPG excretion.

Loraine [20] has recently investigated the effect of the age of the subject and the phase of the cycle on HPG excretion in both nonparous and parous women. For the purposes of the study the results of which are shown in Tables 12-1 and 12-2 the cycle was divided into four phases designated respectively *menstruation, follicular phase, "ovulation,"* and *luteal phase.*

Table 12-1. HPG Excretion in Nonparous Women (from Loraine, [20])

Age	Number of subjects	Number of cycles	HPG excretion during cycle - HMG units/24 hours.			
			Menstruation	Follicular phase	"Ovulation"	Luteal phase
19	2	2	3.7	5.9	5.4	5.0
20-29	4	6	8.4	9.2	12.7	8.9
30-39	2	2	7.9	5.5	7.3	8.0
40-49	1	1	5.0	9.0	13.6	5.2
	9	11	7.0±3.4*	7.9±3.0*	10.5±4.7*	7.7±2.8*

*Standard deviation

Table 12-2. HPG Excretion in Parous Women (from Loraine, [20])

Age	Number of subjects	Number of cycles	HPG excretion during cycle - HMG units/24 hours.			
			Menstruation	Follicular phase	"Ovulation"	Luteal phase
29-39	3	4	14.9	15.0	26.7	11.2
40-49	2	2	7.0	8.2	14.6	6.9
	5	6	12.4±9.9*	12.7±6.5*	20.4±10.4*	9.8±7.8*

*Standard deviation

The period of "ovulation" was considered to extend over five days; it included the day of the midcycle peak of estradiol and estrone with two days on either side of this peak. The mean HPG excretion values together with their standard deviation for the various phases of the cycle are shown in the lowest lines of columns 3 to 6 of the tables.

It should be noted that at all four stages of the cycle the mean HPG readings in parous women were higher than those in nonparous women. When an analysis of variance was performed on the data, it was found that in the nonparous women (Table 12-1) the factor of age was not significant, but that the mean HPG excretion in the ovulatory phase of the cycle was significantly higher than those of the other three phases (P < 0.05). In the parous women (Table 12-2) the factor of age was again insignificant, but a significant difference between phases was found (P < 0.05). It appears reasonable to conclude that this difference results from the fact that the mean HPG excretion in the ovulatory phase of the cycle is considerably higher than that in the other three phases.

Postmenopausal Women

Apostolakis and Loraine [1] studied the HPG excretion in 18 normal ambulant postmenopausal subjects ranging in age from 52 to 77. The mean excretion value was 76.0 HMG units/24 hours and the range (P = 0.95) 35.0 - 158.0 HMG units/24 hours. HPG levels in urine were significantly higher in ambulant subjects than in a group of hospitalized patients suffering from various diseases.

HPG EXCRETION IN PATHOLOGICAL CONDITIONS

Amenorrhea

HPG assays are useful in determining whether the amenorrhea is of pituitary or ovarian origin. In "pituitary" amenorrhea, which results from a disease process affecting the anterior pituitary gland, HPG excretion is very low indeed, and it may not be possible to detect activity even by very sensitive assay methods. In "ovarian" amenorrhea, where the lesion lies in the gonads rather than in the pituitary, HPG excretion is abnormally high and reaches levels similar to those encountered in postmenopausal subjects.

Gemzell, et al. [13], [14] have shown that the most suitable subjects for treatment by human pituitary FSH are those in whom the amenorrhea results from pituitary failure. Patients in whom pretreatment levels are abnormally high do not respond satisfactorily to this form of therapy.

Dysfunctional Uterine Hemorrhage

Urinary HPG assays by reliable methods have not yet been reported in patients with this disease. This is an important field for future investigation.

Dysmenorrhea

Brown, Fotherby, and Loraine [7] have recently studied the HPG excretion in four subjects with this disease. They found levels within the normal range at all stages of the menstrual cycle.

Ovarian Deficiency

It is now well recognized that in patients with primary ovarian failure HPG readings in urine are abnormally high. The condition is well exemplified by the rare disease known as Turner's syndrome (ovarian agenisis), where HPG excretion values are in the range normally encountered in postmenopausal subjects.

Testicular Deficiency

In eunuchoidism due to a lesion of the pituitary, urinary HPG levels are low; if, however, the condition results from testicular disease, the readings are generally high. Apostolakis and Loraine [2] found abnormally high HPG excretion values in five patients suffering from Klinefelter's syndrome; the mean excretion was 40.0 and the highest value obtained 117.0 HMG units/24 hours.

Testicular Tumors

In a recent study in Edinburgh [23] HPG assays have been performed in 20 patients with seminoma and in seven patients with teratoma of the testis; estimations were made following the treatment of these patients by unilateral orchidectomy. In the subjects with seminoma the mean excretion value was 34.0 HMG units/24 hours and the range (P = 0.95) 8.0 to 144.0 HMG units/24 hours; in the patients with teratoma the corresponding figures were 17.0 and 6.0 to 51.0 HMG units/24 hours. The mean excretion values in both seminoma and teratoma were significantly higher than the mean HPG excretion in normal male subjects. They were also significantly higher than that in a group of male subjects of comparable age subjected to unilateral orchidectomy for reasons other than testicular tumor (Loraine, [18]). In view of the observation it appears reasonable to conclude that the operation of unilateral orchidectomy per se was not responsible for the increased pituitary activity found in patients with seminoma and teratoma.

In patients with chorionepithelioma of the testis the gonadotropin output is almost invariably high, but the hormone excreted is human chorionic gonadotropin and not HPG.

Acromegaly

There are few reports in the literature regarding the HPG excretion in patients with this disease. In early cases where the clinical features are those of hyperpituitarism, high excretion values are to be expected. However, in the later stages of the condition, where the symptoms are those of hypopituitarism HPG readings will tend to be below the normal range.

Panhypopituitarism

It is generally agreed that in this condition HPG excretion values are abnormally low, and frequently no activity can be detected even when highly concentrated urinary extracts are assayed by sensitive biological methods such as the mouse uterus test. The presence of gonadotropic activity in the urine of a patient in whom hypopituitarism is suspected makes it necessary to review the diagnosis critically.

Mammary Carcinoma

The clinical value of urinary HPG assays in patients with this disease has been reviewed elsewhere [17], [19]. Assays may be helpful in determining the completeness or otherwise of a surgical hypophysectomy [24] and in predicting the response of postmenopausal subjects with recurrent metastatic mammary carcinoma to treatment with oral stilbestrol [25]. Patients who fail to respond to stilbestrol therapy show significantly higher pretreatment levels of HPG in urine than patients who respond satisfactorily, and it has been postulated [26], that if the HPG excretion before therapy is greater than 55.0 HMG units/24 hours, the patient is unlikely to derive any benefit from stilbestrol and should probably be treated in some other way.

Loraine, et al. [27] have studied the relationship of urinary HPG assays to the treatment of breast cancer by bilateral adrenalectomy and oöphorectomy. They found that such assays were of no value in predicting the response to these operations but that, following adrenalectomy and oöphorectomy, different excretion patterns were found, depending on the response of the patient to this form of treatment. In patients in whom the operations were followed by a remission of disease, excretion values either remained high or tended to rise, while in subjects who failed to respond, the HPG output remained unchanged or tended to fall.

THE EFFECT OF VARIOUS COMPOUNDS ON HPG EXCRETION

This subject has recently been reviewed by Loraine and Bell [21], and the present account is based mainly on their conclusions. Progress in this field will depend on the development of more satisfactory methods for the separate determination of FSH and LH in body fluids and on improved conditions for clinical investigations by means of which subjects can be hospitalized for a relatively long duration, during which time they can be observed throughout adequate control and experimental periods.

The following five groups of substances will be considered: (1) estrogens; (2) androgens; (3) progesterone and progestational compounds; (4) derivatives of dithiocarbamoylhydrazine; and (5) corticosteroids, synthetic analogues, and adrenocorticotropic hormone (ACTH).

Estrogens

Little information is at present available in the literature on the effect of the naturally occurring estrogens on urinary HPG excretion, although it has been claimed that both estradiol and estradiol benzoate are capable of decreasing gonadotropin output in ovariectomized and postmenopausal subjects [35], [41]. On the other hand, potassium estrone sulphate has been shown to be a very weak inhibitor of pituitary gonadotropic function, and Rosemberg and Engel [33] were unable to show any effect on HPG excretion when this compound (2.5 mg/day orally) was administered to a postmenopausal subject for a period of ten days.

It is generally agreed that the synthetic estrogen, stilbestrol, when given orally in sufficiently large dosages, is a potent inhibitor of pituitary gonadotropic function as judged by urinary HPG assays [38], [16]. A typical effect of a relatively large dosage of stilbestrol in a postmenopausal subject with recurrent mammary carcinoma is shown in Fig. 12-1.

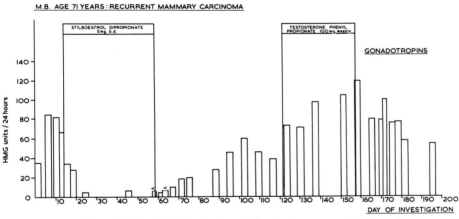

Fig. 12-1. The Effect of Stilbestrol and Testosterone on Urinary HPG Excretion in a Postmenopausal Subject with Mammary Carcinoma.

It should be noted that the drug produced a rapid fall in HPG excretion and that low levels persisted as long as the compound was being administered. After cessation of therapy, readings rose steadily, and within approximately 40 days had reached levels in the same range as those in the pretreatment period.

Androgens

These substances are less active inhibitors of pituitary gonadotropic function than is stilbestrol. Large dosages must be administered for long periods of time before a significant effect on HPG excretion is noted in postmenopausal and ovariectomized subjects [36], [37]. When the dosage is relatively small and the duration of therapy short, there is no effect on HPG output [34], [21].

In Fig. 12-1 is shown the urinary HPG excretion in a postmenopausal subject who received androgen therapy in the form of testosterone phenyl propionate (100 mg/week i. m.). It will be noted that HPG excretion did not fall during the period of drug administration.

Progesterone and Progestational Compounds

Neither Moore, et al. [30] in normally menstruating women, nor Smith and Albert [39], in postmenopausal subjects, could demonstrate any effect of large dosages of progesterone on HPG excretion. It must therefore be assumed that this hormone has little or no pituitary-inhibiting action as far as the gonadotropins are concerned.

Progestational compounds are weak inhibitors of pituitary gonadotropic function, and it is possible that their inhibitory action is due to their conversion in the body to estrogens rather than to the effect of the compounds per se [5]. Both Martin and Cunningham [28], using *nor*ethisterone, and Douglas, et al. [12], using *nor*ethisterone enanthate, have shown that in postmenopausal subjects with recurrent or metastatic mammary carcinoma, HPG excretion is reduced during therapy. Douglas, et al. [12] noted that, in order to produce any appreciable effect on HPG excretion, the progestational compound had to be administered in relatively large amounts, e. g., 200 mg i. m. at weekly intervals. Such treatment did not abolish HPG output but merely reduced it to levels normally encountered in premenopausal subjects. Douglas, et al. [12] found that the drug compared unfavorably with a number of others used routinely in the management of patients with advanced breast cancer and could demonstrate no correlation between the effect on HPG excretion and the response to treatment.

The effect of progestational compounds on hormone excretion in women during reproductive life has been studied by J. B. Brown, et al. [6], [7]. This subject will be discussed on page 207.

Derivatives of Dithiocarbamoylhydrazine

These compounds have been shown by Paget, et al. [32] to be inhibitors of pituitary gonadotropic function in rats, dogs, and monkeys Two such derivatives have recently been investigated for their pituitary-inhibiting properties in human postmenopausal subjects [3].

The compounds studied were:

1.   *Compound 33,828* (Imperial Chemical Industries Ltd.) which is 1-a-methyl-allylthiocarbamoyl-2-methylthiocarbamoyl-hydrazine

$$CH_2 = CH. CH. NH. CS. NH. NH. CS. NH. CH_3$$
$$CH_3$$

2.   *Compound 22,365* (Imperial Chemical Industries Ltd.) which is a less active member of the same chemical series.

It should be emphasized that in contradistinction to many pituitary inhibitors previously described, neither of these compounds is a steroid.

Bell, et al. [3] have shown that in postmenopausal subjects without endocrine disease, these substances decrease urinary HPG excretion but do not affect adrenocortical function as judged by assays of total 17-hydroxycorticosteroids, total 17-ketosteroids, and estrogens. In Fig. 12-2 is shown a typical study with Compound 22,365. In this subject, who was convalescing in the hospital from rheumatic heart disease,

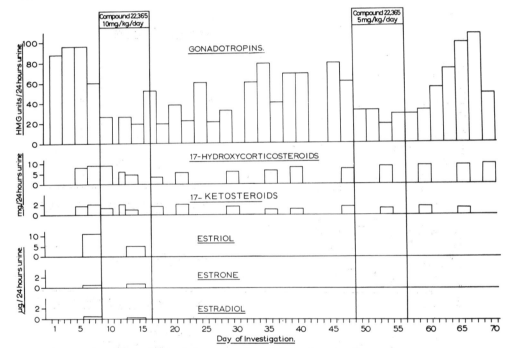

Fig. 12-2. The effect of Compound 22,365 on hormone excretion in a postmenopausal subject (from Bell et al. [4])

the mean HPG level before treatment was 85.0 HMG units/24 hours. Therapy with Compound 22,365 administered orally at dose levels of 10.0 and 5.0 mg/Kg/day produced a marked fall in urinary HPG output, the lowest levels recorded during the two phases of therapy being 19.0 and 18.0 HMG units/24 hours respectively. Approximately 17 days after cessation of treatment at the higher dose level, HPG excretion had reached control values; the corresponding period in the case of the lower dose level was six days.

A similar study with Compound 33,828 in a postmenopausal subject suffering from ischemic heart disease is shown in Fig. 12-3.   The mean HPG output before treatment was 69.0 HMG units/24 hours. Therapy with Compound 33,828 administered orally at the relatively low dose level of 2.5 mg/Kg/day caused a rapid decrease in HPG excretion, the

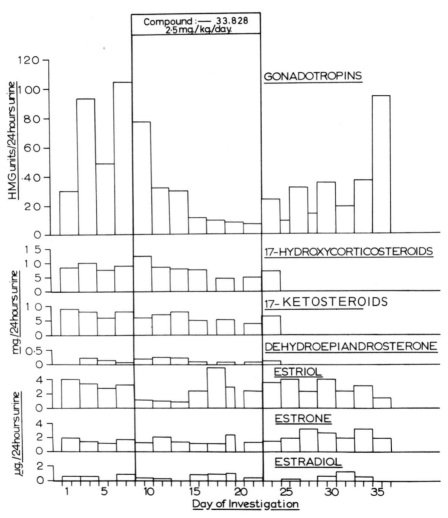

Fig. 12-3.   The effect of Compound 33,828 on hormone excretion in a post-menopausal subject (from Bell, et al. [4])

lowest value recorded during therapy being 7.5 HMG units/24 hours.
After withdrawal of the drug, a rise in HPG output occurred and a
reading similar to those in the control period was found on the 13th
posttreatment day.

The effect of dithiocarbamoylhydrazine derivatives on ovarian and
pituitary function in women during reproductive life has been investigated recently by Bell, et al. [3]. The results are reported on page 210.

Corticosteroids, Synthetic Analogues and ACTH

These substances appear to produce variable effects on urinary
HPG excretion [15], [29], [40]. Increased levels, decreased levels,
and no change in levels have all been reported. Recent investigations
in Edinburgh [11], have shown that a marked rise in HPG excretion can
occur in a proportion of patients being treated for ulcerative colitis and
various types of ileitis by intramuscular ACTH and oral prednisolone;
the rise in HPG levels is most marked in patients responding well to
this form of treatment.

In Fig. 12-4 is shown a study in a male subject with "enterocolitis"
who was treated with ACTH and who responded satisfactorily.

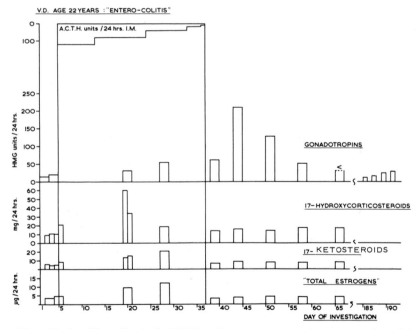

Fig. 12-4. The effect of ACTH on hormone excretion in a male subject
with "enterocolitis."

The marked elevation of HPG levels both during and immediately following therapy should be noted. A reading of 210.0 HMG units/24 hours was encountered seven days after ACTH treatment was stopped; this figure is well above the range normally found in postmenopausal women (see page 186). Readings in the same range as those in the pretreatment period were obtained when the patient was re-investigated approximately 150 days after cessation of therapy.

SUMMARY

1. The main indication for urinary HPG assays in the clinical field is in the differentiation of the various types of gonadal failure.

2. In patients with seminoma and teratoma of the testis, the mean HPG excretion is significantly higher than that in normal male subjects.

3. In patients with recurrent or metastatic mammary carcinoma, urinary HPG assays may be useful in determining the completeness of a hypophysectomy, in predicting the response of patients to oral stilbestrol and in providing information on the course of the disease following bilateral oöphorectomy and adrenalectomy.

4. The synthetic estrogen stilbestrol is a potent depressor of pituitary gonadotropic function in man, while androgenic hormones and progestational compounds are relatively weak pituitary inhibitors.

5. The dithiocarbamoylhydrazine derivatives (Compound 22,365 and 33,828) are nonsteroidal inhibitors of pituitary gonadotropic function in postmenopausal subjects. Neither compound affects adrenocortical function as judged by assays of 17-hydroxycorticosteroids, 17-ketosteroids, and estrogens.

6. In gastrointestinal disorders, both ACTH and corticosteroids are capable of causing a marked rise in urinary HPG levels. Preliminary evidence indicates that increased HPG excretion values are associated with a remission of disease.

REFERENCES

1. Apostolakis, M., and Loraine, J. A. 1960. *J. Clin. Endocrinol.* 20: 1437.

2. Apostolakis, M., and Loraine, J. A. 1960. *Acta Endocrinol. Copenhagen* Suppl. 51: 1089.

3. Bell, E. T., Brown, J. B., Fotherby, K., and Loraine, J. A. 1962. *Lancet* ii: 528.

4. Bell, E. T., Brown, J. B., Fotherby, K., Loraine, J. A., and Robson, J. S. 1962. *J. Endocrinol.* 25: 221.

5. Brown, J. B., and Blair, H. A. F. 1960. *Proc. Roy. Soc. Med.* 53: 433.

6. Brown, J. B., Fotherby, K., and Loraine, J. A. 1960. *Proc. Roy. Soc. Med.* **53**: 431.
7. Brown, J. B., Fotherby, K., and Loraine, J. A. 1962. *J. Endocrinol.* **25**: 331.
8. Brown, J. B., Klopper, A., and Loraine, J. A. 1958. *J. Endocrinol.* **17**: 401.
9. Brown, P. S. 1958. *J. Endocrinol.* **17**: 329.
10. Catchpole, H. R., Greulich, W. W., and Sollenberger, R. T. 1938. *Amer. J. Physiol.* **123**: 32.
11. Crean, G. P., and Loraine, J. A. 1962. Unpublished observations.
12. Douglas, Mary, Loraine, J. A., and Strong, J. A. 1960. *Proc. Roy. Soc. Med.* **53**: 427.
13. Gemzell, C. A., Diczfalusy, E., and Tillinger, K. G. 1958. *J. Clin. Endocrinol.* **18**: 1333.
14. Gemzell, C. A., Dizfalusy, E. and Tillinger, K. G. 1960. In *Ciba Foundation Colloquia on Endocrinology,* London: Churchill, **13**: 191.
15. Lemon, H. M. 1957. *Ann. Intern. Med.* **46**: 457.
16. Loraine, J. A. 1958. *The Clinical Application of Hormone Assay*, Livingstone, Edinburgh, Chap. 2.
17. Loraine, J. A. 1959. In *Cancer*, Butterworth, London, **6**: 160.
18. Loraine, J. A. 1960. In *Ciba Foundation Colloquia on Endocrinology*, Churchill, London, **13**: 233.
19. Loraine, J. A. 1960. *Bull. Soc. Belge. Gynec. Obstet.* **30**: 295.
20. Loraine, J. A. 1962. *Rev. Iber. Endocrinol.* **9**: 7.
21. Loraine, J. A., and Bell, E. T. 1962. In *Proc. Internat. Congr. on Hormonal Steroids* (Milan), Academic Press, New York, In press.
22. Loraine, J. A., and Brown, J. B. 1959. *J. Endocrinol.* **18**: 77.
23. Loraine, J. A., and Schmidt-Elmendorff, H. 1962. In *Modern Trends in Human Reproductive Physiology.*, ed. H. M. Carey, Butterworth, London, 18.
24. Loraine, J. A., and Strong, J. A. 1958. In *Proc. Second Internat. Sympos. on Mammary Cancer*, ed. L. Severi, 119.
25. Loraine, J. A., Strong, J. A., and Douglas, Mary. 1957. *Lancet* ii: 575.
26. Loraine, J. A., Douglas, Mary, Falconer, C. W. A., and Strong, J. A. 1959. In *Extrait de Acta Union Internationale contre le Cancer*, **15**: 1132.
27. Loraine, J. A., Douglas, Mary, Falconer, C. W. A., and Strong, J. A. 1961. *Mem. Soc. Endocrinol.* **10**: 150.
28. Martin, L., and Cunningham, Kathleen. 1961. In *Human Pituitary Gonadotropins*, ed. A. Albert, C. C. Thomas, Springfield, Ill., 226.
29. Mason, H. L., Power, M. H., Rynearson, E. H., Ciaramelli, L. C., Li, C. H., and Evans, H. M. 1948. *J. Clin. Endocrinol.* **8**: 1.
30. Moore, D. J., Roscoe, R. T., Heller, C. G., and Paulsen, C. A. 1961. In *Human Pituitary Gonadotropins*, ed. A. Albert, C. C Thomas, Springfield, Ill., 300.

31. Nathanson, I. T., Towne, L. E., and Aub, J. C. 1941. *Endocrinology* 28: 851.
32. Paget, G. E., Walpole, A. L., and Richardson, D. N. 1961. *Nature,* London 192: 1191.
33. Rosemberg, Eugenia, and Engel, I. 1960. *J. Clin. Endocrinol.* 20: 1576.
34. Rosemberg, Eugenia, and Engel, I. 1961. In *Human Pituitary Gonadotropins,* ed. A. Albert, C. C Thomas, Springfield, Ill., 215.
35. Salmon, U. J., Geist, J. H., and Walter, R. I. 1940. *Proc. Soc. Exper. Biol. N. Y.* 43: 424.
36. Segaloff, A., Gordon, D., Horwitt, B. N., Schlosser, J. V., and Murison, P. J. 1951. *Cancer* 4: 319.
37. Segaloff, A., Horwitt, B. N., Carabasi, R. A., Murison, P. J., and Schlosser, J. V. 1953. *Cancer* 6: 483.
38. Smith, R. A., and Albert, A. 1955. *Proc. Mayo Clin.* 30: 617.
39. Smith, R. A., and Albert, A. 1956. *Proc. Mayo Clin.* 31: 309.
40. Sohval, A. R., and Soffer, L. J. 1951. *J. Clin. Endocrinol.* 11: 677.
41. Tokuyama, I., Leach, R. B., Sheinfield, S., and Maddock, W. O. 1954. *J. Clin. Endocrinol.* 14: 509.

XIII

John A. Loraine, D.Sc., F.R.C.P.E.

SOME CLINICAL APPLICATIONS OF URINARY ESTROGEN ASSAYS IN NONPREGNANT SUBJECTS

INTRODUCTION

Much of the data presented in this chapter has been obtained by the group in Edinburgh, especially by Dr. J. B. Brown, and deals with (1) the excretion of estrogens in normal subjects and (2) estrogen excretion in pathological conditions. In these studies the methods used for the quantitative determination of estrogens in human urine were those developed by Brown [3] and by Brown, et al. [7]. These methods, which are chemical in nature and depend for their final determination on the Kober reaction, measure the three "classical" estrogens— estradiol, estrone, and estriol—and throughout this lecture the term "total estrogen" excretion is used to designate the sum of the excretion values of these three compounds.

ESTROGEN EXCRETION IN NORMAL SUBJECTS

This subject has been previously reviewed (see Loraine [19]), Brown [5], [6], and in the present account an attempt is made to summarize recent developments in this field.

Children

It is generally agreed that the urinary output of estrogens in children and adolescents is relatively low when compared with that of women during reproductive life. Nathanson, et al. [23], using a biological method of assay, found that estrogenic activity could be detected in the urine of boys and girls between the ages of 3 and 7. They noted that the amounts present in the two sexes were approximately equal. In girls, estrogen output increased sharply between the ages of 8 and 11, and after 11 a cyclic pattern of excretion was frequently shown; this cyclic excretion pattern usually preceded the menarche by one or

197

two years. The most detailed study of estrogen excretion in the new-born is that of Tillinger, et al. [25]. These workers, using Brown's method, were unable to detect the presence of estradiol or estriol in the urine of newborn boys but found measurable quantities of estrone.

Normal Men

Small but readily detectable quantities of estrogens have been demonstrated in male urine by bioassay techniques. The main site of production is almost certainly the adrenal cortex, although the testes may contribute. In a study by Brown [4], estrogen assays were per-formed in 29 normal male subjects ranging in age from 20 to 50 years. The mean total estrogen excretion was 10.3 μg/24 hours and the values ranged from 6.0 to 17.8 μg/24 hours.

Normally Menstruating Women

The characteristic pattern of estrogen excretion in the ovulatory menstrual cycle is shown in Fig. 13-1. This figure, which was com-piled from observations made in 16 subjects aged from 18 to 41 years, shows the mean excretion of the three "classical" estrogens together with their arithmetic ranges for the various stages of the cycle.

During the first seven to ten days of the cycle, the output of the three estrogens is low, and the mean figure for total estrogen excre-tion is below 20.0 μg/24 hours. Levels start to rise on or about the seventh day of the cycle and reach a well-defined maximum—the *ovulation peak*—from day 12 to day 14, at which stage the mean total estrogen excretion exceeds 50.0 μg/24 hours. After ovulation there is a rapid fall in excretion values for all three estrogens; this is succeeded by a second rise—the *luteal maximum*—which occurs from the nine-teenth to the twenty-first day and persists until shortly before the on-set of the next menstrual period. Immediately prior to menstruation, estrogen excretion falls, but the lowest levels throughout the whole cycle are frequently found some days after the onset of bleeding.

The relationship between the ovulatory peak of estrogens and the HPG peak has been discussed elsewhere (see p. 184). It will be remem-bered [9] that the midcycle estrogen peak either coincided with the HPG peak or preceded it by an interval of up to three days.

Menopausal and Postmenopausal Women

Estrogens can be detected in relatively small quantities in the urine of menopausal and postmenopausal women, and it is presumed that the main source of production is the adrenal cortex. One of the most careful studies on this subject is that of McBride [21], who esti-mated the estrogen excretion twice weekly for six to eight weeks in seven subjects in whom the menopause had occurred from two to 26 years previously. The mean total estrogen excretion was 5.8 μg/24 hours and the values ranged from 3.1 to 8.1 μg/24 hours. No correlation could be demonstrated between the estrogen output and the time after the menopause, and there was no evidence of a cyclic pattern of excretion.

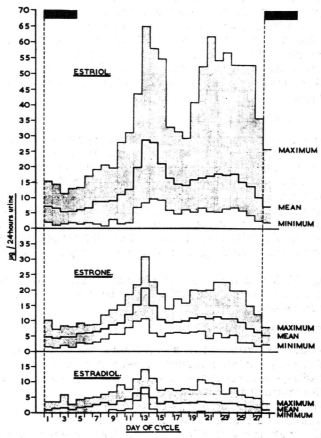

Fig. 13-1. Estrogen excretion during the normal menstrual cycle (from Brown [5]).   ▬▬▬ menstrual bleeding

ESTROGEN EXCRETION IN PATHOLOGICAL CONDITIONS

Disorders of Menstruation

Amenorrhea

In patients with this condition, estrogen excretion is generally low and is frequently within the range normally encountered in postmenopausal subjects. Low values are found irrespective of whether the amenorrhea is primary or secondary or is of ovarian or pituitary origin. In a series of eight subjects reported by Brown, et al. [8] and classified as "menopause praecox" the mean total estrogen excretion was 6.3 μg/24 hours and the range was from 1.8 to 10.0 μg/24 hours.

In three subjects with primary amenorrhea due to a congenital absence of the uterus, Brown, et al. [8] observed a cyclical pattern of urinary estrogen excretion with levels in the same range as those in the ovulatory menstrual cycle (see Fig. 13-1). These findings indicate that normal ovarian activity can occur in the absence of the target organ, the uterus.

Anovulatory Menstrual Cycles

According to Brown, et al. [8] the estrogen excretion in anovulatory menstrual cycles shows two main characteristics.

1. Excretion values remain more or less constant between episodes of bleeding. This is in marked contrast to the ovular menstrual cycle, in which a rhythmic pattern of excretion is found.

2. Readings are generally higher than those in patients with complete amenorrhea and an atrophic endometrium. In a series of 11 anovulatory cycles in six subjects, Brown, et al. [8] reported a mean total estrogen excretion of 18.2 μg/24 hours and a range of 9.0 to 33.0 μg/24 hours.

In Fig. 13-2 is shown the estrogen excretion in an anovular followed by an ovular menstrual cycle. The contrast between the two cycles should be noted.

Cystic Glandular Hyperplasia

The characteristic features in patients with this disease are:

1. The very variable pattern of estrogen excretion. In some subjects readings remain more or less constant, while in others considerable fluctuations in levels occur.

2. The fact that very high readings—sometimes up to 100 g total estrogens per 24 hours—can be obtained.

3. The lack of correlation between the estrogen output and the duration and severity of the bleeding.

In Fig. 13-3, which is taken from a paper by Brown, et al. [8], the total estrogen excretion remained relatively constant throughout the period of study, the level being generally above 30.0 μg/24 hours. The constancy of the levels during the relatively protracted phase of bleeding should be noted.

Stein-Leventhal Syndrome

Little reliable information is at present available on the estrogen excretion in patients with this disease. In a subject studied recently in Edinburgh, estrogen levels before therapy were in the range normally

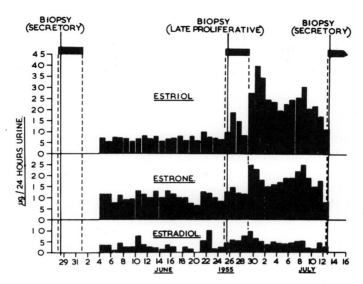

Fig. 13-2. Estrogen excretion in an anovular followed by an ovular menstrual cycle (from Brown et al. [8]).   ▬▬▬ phase of bleeding

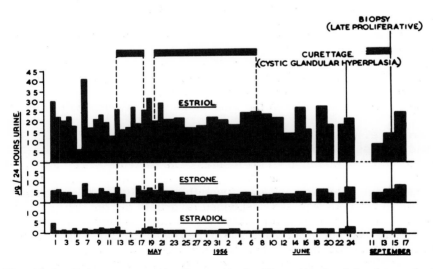

Fig. 13-3. Estrogen excretion in a patient with cystic glandular hyperplasis (from Brown, et al. [8]).   ▬▬▬ phase of bleeding

encountered in postmenopausal women. Following treatment with the nonsteroidal compound Clomiphene (MRL-41), two ovulatory menstrual cycles occurred in which the estrogen excretion was within normal limits for women during reproductive life. This finding supports the view of Greenblatt, et al. [17], that Clomiphene is capable of inducing ovulation in a proportion of patients suffering from the Stein-Leventhal syndrome. (see Chapter 7).

Ovarian Tumors

In patients with *granulosa cell tumor* of the ovaries, estrogen levels in urine are generally abnormally high. Removal of the tumor causes a sharp fall in estrogen excretion, while the presence of re- currences in the contralateral ovary is indicated by a rise in output. Sometimes, however, elevated estrogen levels in urine are not found in patients with functioning ovarian tumors; in two such subjects with combined granulosal and thecal cell tumors investigated by Brown, et al. [8] the mean total estrogen excretion was only 13.0 μg/24 hours.

Mammary Carcinoma

Estrogen assays have been performed in patients with recurrent or metastatic mammary carcinoma for three main reasons:

1. To determine whether any abnormality of estrogen production or metabolism exists in patients with this disease.

2. To attempt to predict by such assays the response of patients to various forms of therapy.

3. To study the effect of various forms of hormonal treatment on the estrogen output.

In spite of a great amount of work in various centers the results from the clinical point of view have been disappointing, and it can be stated that, at the time of writing, urinary estrogen assays have proved of little or no value in the management of patients with this disease.

Strong, et al. [24] studied the estrogen excretion in 13 patients who had previously undergone bilateral adrenalectomy and bilateral oöphorectomy for mammary carcinoma. The patients were classified into two clinical groups—"success" or "failure"—according to their response to the operation. It was found that the pattern of estrogen excretion in patients who had responded favorably did not differ from that in patients who showed no improvement after removal of both adrenals and ovaries. Bulbrook and Greenwood [10] investigated the effect of bilateral oöphorectomy, bilateral adrenalectomy, and hypophysectomy on estrogen excretion in patients with mammary carcinoma. They found that estrogen excretion generally continued unchanged after oöphorectomy and that, in a proportion of cases, it was not completely abolished by subsequent adrenalectomy. Persist- ence of estrogen production, as judged by the findings on urinary assay, was also demonstrated in postmenopausal and oöphorectomized patients subjected to hypophysectomy.

Prostatic Carcinoma

Bulbrook, et al. [11], [12] compared the estrogen excretion in 18 subjects with untreated prostatic carcinoma with that of a series of 22 male subjects hospitalized for reasons other than cancer. No differences between the two groups were noted either in terms of the total estrogen output or in the relative proportion of the various estrogens excreted. When the patients were treated with the synthetic estrogen stilbestrol, only estrone and estriol could be measured because the compound interferred with the estimation of estradiol. In the majority of subjects, stilbestrol caused a fall in urinary estrogen excretion, and reactivation of the tumor was associated with a rise in estrogen output. Accordingly, it was concluded that a positive correlation existed between tumor growth and estrogen excretion.

Adrenocortical Tumors and Adrenocortical Hyperplasia

In the rare feminizing type of adrenocortical tumor, abnormally high amounts of urinary estrogen are generally found [14], [20]. In a male patient studied by Brown [6], a total estrogen output of 1318.0 μg/ 24 hours was found; levels dropped to normal on removal of the tumor.

Eberlein, et al. [15] have shown that in children and young women suffering from adrenocortical hyperplasia, estriol levels in urine are generally above the normal range. In all subjects a marked decrease in estriol excretion occurred when the patients were treated with cortisone or with synthetic analogues.

Testicular Tumors

Information on the pattern of estrogen excretion in patients with testicular tumors is very scanty. Hamburger [18], using bioassay methods, has claimed that the estrogen output in cases of seminoma is generally within normal limits, while high readings are to be expected in patients with chorionepithelioma. In a recent study conducted in Edinburgh, abnormally high total estrogen excretion values were found in a proportion of patients with seminoma of the testis. These readings fell abruptly when the tumor was treated by unilateral orchidectomy.

Myocardial Infarction

Estrogen metabolism in patients with this disease had been studied by Bauld, et al. [1], who administered small doses of estradiol to male subjects convalescent in the hospital after a recent myocardial infarction and compared their findings with those in a group of healthy men of comparable age. They found that the amounts of total estrogen excreted in the urine as a percentage of the dose administered was the same in the two groups, but that the patients with myocardial infarction excreted relatively more of the estrogen as estriol than the control group.

Liver Disease

Many observations both in man and in experimental animals indicate that the liver is the main organ responsible for the metabolism of the estrogens. In addition, it has been widely believed that in patients with liver disease certain clinical features such as gynaecomastia, testicular atrophy, spider naevi, and palmar erythema result from the presence of abnormally large quantities of circulating estrogens.

The most detailed investigation so far reported on endogenous estrogen excretion in patients with chronic liver damage is probably that of Cameron [13], who studied 12 such subjects. He found an abnormally high total estrogen excretion in only two cases; in the remainder the figures were within the normal range. Bloomburg, et al. [2] found that the mean estrogen excretion in patients with cirrhosis of the liver was higher than that in control subjects and that the increase was mainly in the estriol fraction; a similar observation has been made by Brown [5].

A number of studies have been performed on the metabolic fate of injected estrogens in patients with hepatic cirrhosis [22]. It is generally agreed that impairment of estrogen metabolism is indicative of a very poor prognosis, as this abnormality is not usually found unless the patient is in an almost moribund condition.

It is obvious that much further work on the relationship of estrogen excretion to hepatic disease is necessary. The field may well be a promising one for future investigations.

Hypertrophic Pulmonary Osteoarthropathy

Ginsburg and Brown [16] have recently studied the estrogen excretion in 11 males with this disease and have compared their results in patients with carcinoma of the bronchus without arthropathy and in healthy subjects. They found that the mean estrogen excretion in the patients with hypertrophic pulmonary osteoarthropathy was more than double that of the other two groups. A few of the patients in the series showed the presence of gynecomastia, but no correlation could be demonstrated between the presence of this complication and the urinary estrogen output. The cause of the raised estrogen output in patients with this disease is at present completely unknown, and the problem remains one for future elucidation.

SUMMARY

1. Reliable figures are now available for the excretion of estrogens during the normal menstrual cycle. Readings are low in the early follicular phase and just prior to the onset of menstruation; peaks of excretion occur at midcycle and during the luteal phase.

2. The estrogen excretion in men, postmenopausal women, and children is low and is mainly of adrenal origin.

3. In abnormal gynecological conditions, estrogen assays may be of diagnostic value in anovulatory menstrual cycles and in cystic glandular hyperplasia. Abnormally high readings are generally found in functioning ovarian tumors.

4. Estrogen assays by currently available techniques are of little value in the management of patients with mammary and prostatic carcinoma.

5. Estrogen levels in urine are generally above the normal range in patients with adrenocortical hyperplasia and feminizing tumors of the adrenal cortex.

6. In male patients with hypertrophic pulmonary osteoarthropathy, urinary estrogen excretion values are significantly higher than in healthy male subjects.

REFERENCES

1. Bauld, W. S., Givner, M. L., and Milne, I. G. 1957. *Canad. J. Biochem. Physiol.* 25: 1277.
2. Bloomberg, B. M., Miller, K., Keeley, K. J., and Higginson, J. 1958. *J. Endocrinol.* 17: 182.
3. Brown, J. B. 1955. *Biochem. J.* 60: 185.
4. Brown, J. B. 1955. *Mem. Soc. Endocrinol.* 3: 1.
5. Brown, J. B. 1960. In *Clinical Endocrinology,* Grune & Stratton, Inc., New York, 684.
6. Brown, J. B. 1960. In *Advances in Clinical Chemistry*, Academic Press, New York, 3: 157.
7. Brown, J. B., Bulbrook, R. D., and Greenwood, F. C. 1957. *J. Endocrinol.* 16: 49.
8. Brown, J. B., Kellar, R. J., and Matthew, G. D. 1959. *J. Obstet. Gynaec. Brit. Emp.* 66: 177.
9. Brown, J. B., Klopper, A., and Loraine, J. A. 1958. *J. Endocrinol.* 17: 401.
10. Bulbrook, R. D., and Greenwood, F. C. 1957. *Brit. Med. J.* 1: 662.
11. Bulbrook, R. D., Franks, L. M., and Greenwood, F. C. 1959. *Acta. Endocrinol.* Copenhagen, 31: 481.
12. Bulbrook, R. D., Franks, L. M., and Greenwood, F. C. 1959. *Brit. J. Cancer* 13: 45.

13. Cameron, C. B. 1957. *J. Endocrinol.* 15: 199.
14. Diczfalusy, E., and Luft, R. 1952. *Acta Endocrinol.* Copenhagen, 9: 327.
15. Eberlein, W. R., Bongiovanni, A. M., and Francis, C. M. 1958. *J. Clin. Endocrinol.* 18: 1274.
16. Ginsburg, Jean, and Brown, J. B. 1961. *Lancet* ii: 1274.
17. Greenblatt, R. B., Mahesh, V. B., and Roy, S. 1962. In *Proc. Internat. Congr. Hormonal Steroids:* (Milan) No. 173.
18. Hamburger, C. 1938. In *Les Hormones Sexuelles,* ed. L. Brouha, Hermann, Paris, 345.
19. Loraine, J. A. 1958. *The Clinical Application of Hormone Assay.* Livingstone, Edinburgh, Chap. 9.
20. Luft, R., and Sjögren, B. 1949. *Acta Endocrinol.* Copenhagen, 3: 342.
21. McBride, J. B. 1957. *J. Clin. Endocrinol.* 17: 1440.
22. May, J. A., and Stimmel, B. F. 1955. *Calif. Med.* 82: 171.
23. Nathanson, I. T., Towne, L. E., and Aub, J. C. 1941. *Endocrinology* 28: 85.
24. Strong, J. A., Brown, J. B., Bruce, J., Douglas, Mary, Klopper, A., and Loraine, J. A. 1956. *Lancet* ii: 955.
25. Tillinger, K. G., Diczfalusy, E., and Westman, A. 1957. *Acta Endocrinol.* Copenhagen Suppl. 31: 47.

XIV

John A. Loraine, D.Sc., F.R.C.P.E.

THE EFFECT OF CONTRACEPTIVE DRUGS ON HORMONE EXCRETION DURING THE MENSTRUAL CYCLE

INTRODUCTION

This chapter deals with two groups of compounds:

1. The *progestational compounds nor*ethisterone (17α-ethynyl-19-*nor*testosterone) and its acetate. Compounds of this general structure have been widely used as contraceptive agents and their clinical effects are now well documented [12], [13].

2. The *dithiocarbamoylhydrazine derivative,* Compound 33,828 (see Chapter XII).

The present account, which is based on publications by Brown, et al. [5], [6], Loraine [10], and Bell, et al. [1], is concerned with the effects of these substances on the urinary excretion of estrogens, pregnanediol, pregnanetriol, and human pituitary gonadotropins (HPG) in women during reproductive life. In these studies estriol, estrone, and estradiol were measured by the methods of Brown [3] and Brown, et al. [4]; pregnanediol and pregnanetriol were determined respectively by the methods of Klopper, et al. [8] and Fotherby and Love [8], while for the estimation of HPG in urine the method of Loraine and Brown [11] was used.

THE EFFECT OF NORETHISTERONE AND ITS ACETATE

In Fig. 14-1 are shown the findings in a subject with dysmenorrhoea but with previously regular 27-day menstrual cycles. This subject was studied throughout three cycles, in the second of which she received *nor*ethisterone (20 mg/day orally) from the 5th to the 29th day. In the first and third cycles no treatment was given.

In the first cycle, menstruation lasted for six days and the subject experienced severe dysmenorrhea from the 22nd to the 25th day. The pattern of hormone excretion indicated the presence of a normal ovula-

tory menstrual cycle; the absence of an HPG peak at midcycle should
be noted.

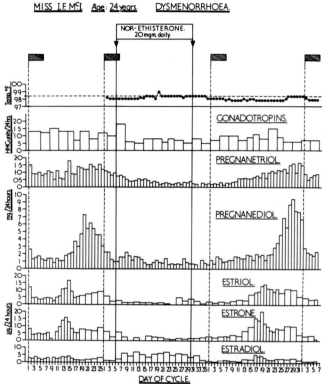

Fig. 14-1.   Hormone excretion in a subject with dysmenorrhea treated
with *nor*ethisterone.   Hatched areas indicate menstrual bleeding.
(From Brown, et al. [6].)

    In the second cycle, menstruation also lasted for six days; pre-
menstrual dysmenorrhea was absent and the compound produced a well-
marked hyperthermic effect.   Pregnanetriol excretion was depressed
during treatment with *nor*ethisterone, and the rise in pregnanediol excretion, which normally occurs in the luteal phase of the cycle was
absent.   Estrogen output remained low throughout, and the peaks of
excretion which normally occur at midcycle and in the luteal phase
were absent.   HPG was present in urine at all stages of the cycle, the
highest reading being immediately after the cessation of menstruation.
    In the third cycle the findings were similar to those in the first.
Menstrual bleeding lasted for six days and there was again severe
dysmenorrhea towards the end of the cycle.   The excretion of estrogens
and pregnanediol was within the normal range, and urinary pregnanetriol readings showed a steady rise throughout the cycle.   The HPG

output varied from 8.0 -15.0 HMG units/24 hours without a definite peak of excretion at midcycle.

A similar study to that in Fig. 14-1 is shown in Fig. 14-2.

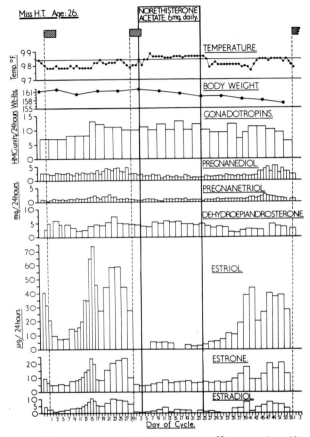

Fig. 14-2. Hormone excretion in a normally menstruating subject treated with *nor*ethisterone acetate. Hatched areas indicate menstrual bleeding. (From Loraine [10].)

This subject with previously regular 30-day menstrual cycles and without dysmenorrhea was observed over a period of time equivalent to three cycles. The initial "control" cycle was ovulatory in character. In the second cycle, *nor*ethisterone acetate (6 mg/day orally) was administered from the 4th to the 25th day. After cessation of therapy, a withdrawal bleeding did not occur but, in spite of this fact, the subject in the last four weeks of the study showed the findings characteristic of an ovular menstrual cycle.

In the second cycle, the normal luteal phase rise in urinary pregnanediol did not occur, and the midcycle and luteal phase peaks of estrogen excretion were absent. Nevertheless, urinary HPG output
continued at levels comparable to those in the two cycles in which
treatment with the progestational compound was not given.
Comment. The results in Figs. 14-1 and 14-2 indicate that *nor*ethisterone and its acetate can inhibit ovulation as judged by steroid excretion without affecting urinary HPG excretion. This finding is compatible with the view that these compounds exert their effects by a
direct action on the ovaries rather than through the pituitary. It
should, however, be emphasized that the bioassay method employed
for the determination of HPG, i. e., the mouse uterus test, measures
both FSH and LH [9], [14], and that therefore the data reported herein
do not exclude the possibility of a differential action on one or other of
the pituitary gonadotropins.

THE EFFECT OF THE DITHIOCARBAMOYLHYDRAZINE DERIVATIVE COMPOUND 33,828

In Fig. 14-3 the findings in a normally menstruating subject, aged
28, are shown.

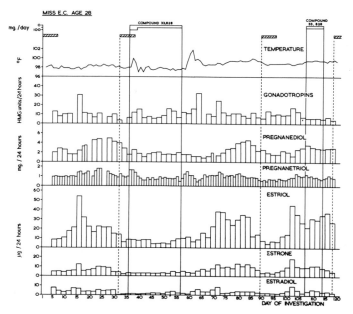

Fig. 14-3. Hormone excretion in a normally menstruating subject treated
with Compound 33,828 (Imperial Chemical Industries Ltd.). Hatched
areas indicate menstrual bleeding. (From Bell, et al. [1].)

The study was conducted over a period of 120 days. In the first cycle the compound was not administered. In the second cycle the drug was given orally from day 5 to day 25, first at a dose level of 100 mg/day and subsequently, because of complaints of nausea, lethargy, and drowsiness, at a dose level of 50 mg/day. In the last cycle the compound was administered in the luteal phase only from day 19 to day 25. The following points should be noted:

1. The first cycle was of a normal ovulatory character.
2. During the administration of the Compound in the second cycle, the luteal phase rise in pregnanediol and the midcycle and luteal phase peaks of estrogen excretion were absent. Nevertheless, HPG excretion continued at levels comparable to those in the control cycle.
3. When administration of the Compound was stopped, menstrual bleeding did not take place for a further 32 days, during which time a normal ovulatory cycle occurred.
4. In the last cycle when the Compound was administered from day 19 to day 25, no effect on luteal function was observed.

Comment. The data shown in Fig. 14-3 indicate that the dithiocarbamoylhydrazine derivative, Compound 33,828, is capable of inhibiting ovulation, as judged by steroid excretion, without affecting HPG output. In this respect it resembles the progestational compound *nor*ethisterone and its acetate (see p. 210), and the inference is that both groups of compounds produce their effects by a direct action on the ovaries rather than through the pituitary. It should, however, be emphasized that the dosage of Compound 33,828 administered was relatively small, and that when larger dosages are given to postmenopausal women (see p. 191), inhibition of pituitary gonadotropic function occurs and HPG excretion in urine is decreased [2].

In the case of *nor*ethisterone and its acetate, the progestational and estrogenic effects of the compounds usually result in a withdrawal bleeding a few days after cessation of thereapy. However, Compound 33,828 possesses no such hormonal properties, and for this reason bleeding does not occur after treatment is withdrawn. Preliminary evidence [1] indicates that the suppression of ovarian function produced by the dithiocarbamoylhydrazine derivative is temporary and completely reversible. However, much work will be necessary before any definite conclusions can be drawn regarding its long-term effects on the ovary and the pituitary.

REFERENCES

1. Bell, E. T., Brown, J. B., Fotherby, K., and Loraine, J. A. 1962. *Lancet.* ii: 528.
2. Bell, E. T., Brown, J. B., Fotherby, K., Loraine, J. A., and Robson, J. S. 1962. *J. Endocrinol.* 25: 221.

3. Brown, J. B.   1955. *Biochem. J.* 60: 185.
4. Brown, J. B., Bulbrook, R. D., and Greenwood, F. C.   1957. *J. Endocrinol.* 16: 49.
5. Brown, J. B., Fotherby, K., and Loraine, J. A.   1960. *Proc. Roy. Soc. Med.* 53: 431.
6. Brown, J. B., Fotherby, K., and Loraine, J. A.   1962. *J. Endocrinol.* 25: 331.
7. Fotherby, K., and Love, D. N.   1960. *J. Endocrinol.* 20: 157.
8. Klopper, A., Michie, Eileen A., and Brown, J. B.   1955. *J. Endocrinol.* 12: 209.
9. Loraine, J. A.   1958. *The Clinical Application of Hormone Assay,* Livingstone, Edinburgh, Chap. 2.
10. Loraine, J. A.   1962. *Rev. Iber. Endocrinol.* 9: 7.
11. Loraine, J. A., and Brown, J. B.   1959. *J. Endocrinol.* 18: 77.
12. Mears, Eleanor.   1961. *Brit. Med. J.* 2: 1179.
13. Pincus, G., Rock, J., Garcia, C. R., Rice-Wray, E., Paniagua, M., and Rodriguez, I.   1958. *Amer. J. Obstet and Gynec.* 75: 1333.
14. Schmidt-Elmendorff, H., Loraine, J. A., and Bell, E. T.   1962. *J. Endocrinol.* 24: 349.

AUTHOR INDEX

213

SUBJECT INDEX

A

221